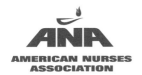

AMERICAN NURSES
ASSOCIATION

Scope AND
Standards
OF PRACTICE

Nursing Informatics: Scope and Standards of Practice

Second Edition

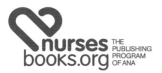

nurses
books.org
THE PUBLISHING PROGRAM OF ANA

American Nurses Association
Silver Spring, Maryland
2015

The American Nurses Association (ANA) is a national professional association. This publication, *Nursing Informatics: Scope and Standards of Practice, Second Edition,* reflects the thinking of the practice specialty of nursing informatics on various issues and should be reviewed in conjunction with state board of nursing policies and practices. State law, rules, and regulations govern the practice of nursing, while *Nursing Informatics: Scope and Standards of Practice, Second Edition,* guides informatics nurses in the application of their professional skills and responsibilities.

The American Nurses Association is the only full-service professional organization representing the interests of the nation's 3.1 million registered nurses through its constituent/state nurses associations and its organizational affiliates. The ANA advances the nursing profession by fostering high standards of nursing practice, promoting the rights of nurses in the workplace, projecting a positive and realistic view of nursing, and by lobbying the Congress and regulatory agencies on healthcare issues affecting nurses and the public.

American Nurses Association
8515 Georgia Avenue, Suite 400
Silver Spring, MD 20910-3492
1-800-274-4ANA
http://www.Nursingworld.org

Published by Nursesbooks.org
The Publishing Program of ANA
http://www.Nursesbooks.org/

ISBN-13: 978-1-55810-579-9   SAN: 851-3481   4/2015R

First printing: November 2014.
Second printing: April 2015.

Contents

Contributors

Work Group Members

William Donovan, MA, RN, Chairperson

Linda Dietrich, MSN, RN-BC, PMP, CPHQ

Sandra Blair Ekimoto, MBA, BS, RN

Paulette Fraser, MS, RN-BC

Sharon Giarrizzo-Wilson, MS, RN-BC, CNOR

Linda Harrington, PhD, DNP, RN-BC, CNS, CPHQ, CENP, CPHIMS, FHIMSS

Luann Whittenburg, PhD, RN-BC, FNP-BC, CPHQ, CPHIMS

Kathleen "Katie" Hoy Johnson, DNP, RN-BC, NCSN

Mary Lynn McHugh, PhD, RN

Leigh Ann Chandler Poole, PhD, RN, FNP-BC, CRNP, CTCP, CTC

Cheryl D. Parker, PhD, RN-BC, FHIMSS

Troy Seagondollar, MSN-I, RN-BC

Nadia Sultana, DNP, MBA, RN-BC

Advisory Group Members

Theresa L. Calderone, EdD, Med, MSN, RN-BC

Lory J. Maddox, MSN, MBA, RN

Susan A. Matney, MSN, RN, FAAN

Darla Shehy, MSN, RN

Rhonda Struck, BSN, RN, MS

American Nurses Association Staff

Carol Bickford, PhD, RN-BC, CPHIMS, FAAN

Maureen Cones, Esq.

Eric Wurzbacher, BA

Yvonne Humes, MSA

About the American Nurses Association

The American Nurses Association (ANA) is the only full-service professional organization representing the interests of the nation's 3.1 million registered nurses through its constituent/state nurses associations and its organizational affiliates. The ANA advances the nursing profession by fostering high standards of nursing practice, promoting the rights of nurses in the workplace, projecting a positive and realistic view of nursing, and by lobbying the Congress and regulatory agencies on healthcare issues affecting nurses and the public.

About Nursesbooks.org, The Publishing Program of ANA

Nursesbooks.org publishes books on ANA core issues and programs, including ethics, leadership, quality, specialty practice, advanced practice, and the profession's enduring legacy. Best known for the foundational documents of the profession on nursing ethics, scope and standards of practice, and social policy, Nursesbooks.org is the publisher for the professional, career-oriented nurse, reaching and serving nurse educators, administrators, managers, and researchers as well as staff nurses in the course of their professional development.

The Scope of Nursing Informatics Practice

Introduction

The American Nurses Association (ANA) identified nursing informatics as a nursing specialty in 1992. The first scope of practice statement for this specialty, *Scope of Practice for Nursing Informatics*, was published in 1994, followed by the 1995 release of an accompanying resource, *Standards of Practice for Nursing Informatics*. Those early publications were replaced in 2001 by the *Scope and Standards of Nursing Informatics Practice*, which combined both the scope and standards of practice into one document and created an enhanced and more robust definition of nursing informatics to reflect the contemporary healthcare informatics environment. The 2008 *Nursing Informatics: Scope and Standards of Practice* followed with a slightly revised specialty definition of nursing informatics and inclusion of an expanded presentation of compe tencies for the informatics nurse and informatics nurse specialist.

The publication of this second edition of *Nursing Informatics: Scope and Standards of Practice* is the culmination of an 18-month-long intensive professional review and revision initiative hosted by ANA. Dedicated workgroup members with more than 280 person years of nursing and informatics expertise met at least twice a month via telephone conference calls from April 2013 until the final draft was completed in July 2014. Weekly meetings became the norm as the workgroup members evaluated every response received from the 30-day public comment period. The final draft completed a two-step ANA review process with examination by the ANA Committee on Nursing Practice Standards and final approval by the Board of Directors.

Definition of Nursing Informatics

Nursing informatics (NI) is the specialty that integrates nursing science with multiple information and analytical sciences* to identify, define, manage, and

---

* A listing of sciences that integrate with nursing informatics includes, but is not limited to: computer science, cognitive science, the science of terminologies and taxonomies (including naming and coding conventions), information management, library science, heuristics, archival science, and mathematics.

communicate data, information, knowledge, and wisdom in nursing practice. NI supports nurses, consumers, patients, the interprofessional healthcare team, and other stakeholders in their decision-making in all roles and settings to achieve desired outcomes. This support is accomplished through the use of information structures, information processes, and information technology.

The nursing informatics specialty and its constituent members contribute to achieving the goal of improving the health of populations, communities, groups, families, and individuals. Supporting activities include, but are not limited to, the identification of issues and the design, development, and implementation of effective informatics solutions and technologies within the clinical, administrative, educational, and research domains of practice.

Metastructures, Concepts, and Tools of Nursing Informatics

Metastructures: Data, Information, Knowledge, and Wisdom

In the mid-1980s, Blum (1986) introduced the concepts of data, information, and knowledge as a framework for understanding clinical information systems and their impact on health care. Blum classified clinical information systems according to the three types of objects that these systems processed: data, information, and knowledge. Blum noted that the classification was artificial, with no clear boundaries, although the categories did represent a scale of increasing complexity.

In 1989, Graves and Corcoran built on these ideas in their seminal study of nursing informatics using the concepts of data, information, and knowledge. They contributed two general principles to NI: a definition of nursing informatics that has been widely accepted in the field, and an information management model that identified data, information, and knowledge as key components of NI practice (Figure 1).

Drawing from Blum's 1986 work, Graves and Corcoran defined the three concepts as follows:

■ *Data* are discrete entities that are described objectively without interpretation.

■ *Information* is data that have been interpreted, organized, or structured.

■ *Knowledge* is information that is synthesized so that relationships are identified and formalized.

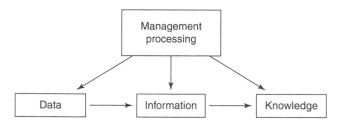

Figure 1. Conceptual Framework for the Study of Nursing Knowledge
Source: Graves & Corcoran (1989). Reprinted with permission of the publisher.

Data, information, and knowledge are of value to nurses in all areas of practice. Data may be obtained from multiple sources; the data are processed into information and then into knowledge. For example, data derived from direct care of an individual can be compiled across disease states and then aggregated for decision-making by nurses, nurse administrators, or other health professionals. Further aggregation can encompass geographical populations. Nurse educators can create case studies using these data, and nurse researchers can access the aggregated data for systematic study.

The appropriate use of knowledge involves the integration of empirical, ethical, personal, and aesthetic knowledge into actions. The individual must apply a high level of empirical knowledge in understanding the current situation, apply a professional value system in considering possible actions, be able to predict the potential outcome of these actions with a high level of accuracy, and then have the means to carry out the selected action in the given environment.

Wisdom is defined as the appropriate use of knowledge to manage and solve human problems. It consists of knowing when and how to apply knowledge to deal with complex problems or specific human needs (Nelson & Joos, 1989; Nelson, 2002; Nelson & Staggers, 2014). Whereas knowledge focuses on what is known, wisdom focuses on the appropriate application of that knowledge and an appreciation of the consequences of selected actions. For example, a knowledge base may include several options for managing an anxious family; wisdom involves nursing judgment about which of these options is most appropriate for a specific family, and use of that option in the care of that family.

An example can help distinguish data, information, knowledge, and wisdom. If a nurse receives the list of numbers, 28, 68, 94, 98, and 110, those raw numbers are certainly data, but they are meaningless. If, however, the numbers are ordered, structured, and identified as follows: T 98°, P 94, R 28, and BP 110/68, the nurse recognizes this series as measurements of vital signs and will regard those numbers as information. Nevertheless, the nurse must be able to place these measures in the context of a particular patient's situation in order to interpret the meaning of those values. If these vital signs were obtained from a newborn, they mean one thing; if they were obtained from an adult, they have a very different meaning. The nurse's knowledge of normal vital sign values for different types of patients, and the condition of the patient from whom the numbers were obtained, provide a context within which the nurse can interpret the information. Then the nurse will know if the numbers represent a normal, expected result or an abnormal, even pathological result. The numbers must be placed in a particular context so that the nurse can take appropriate clinical action, thereby demonstrating "knowledge-in-use" or wisdom.

Figure 2 builds on the work of Graves and Corcoran by depicting the relationship of data, information, knowledge, and wisdom. As data are

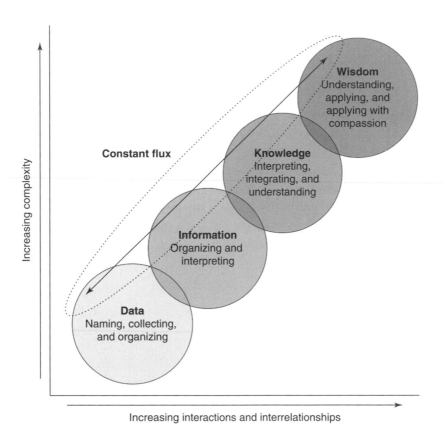

Figure 2. The Relationship of Data, Information, Knowledge, and Wisdom

(Copyright 2002 Ramona Nelson, Ramona Nelson Consulting. All rights reserved. Reprinted with permission.)

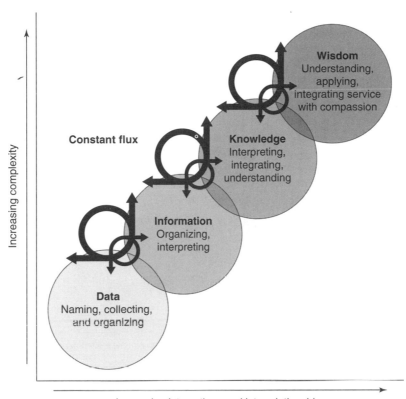

Figure 3. Revised Data Information Knowledge Wisdom (DIKW) Model—2013 Version

transformed into information and information into knowledge, each level increases in complexity and requires greater application of human intellect. The x-axis represents interactions within and the interrelationships between the concepts as one moves from data to wisdom; the y-axis represents the increasing complexity of the concepts.

Figure 3 reflects Nelson's recent evolution of her 2002 model depicting the dynamic interactivity of the inter- and intra-environmental factors that influence the movement across and within the data-to-wisdom continuum.

In a newly published model, Nelson identifies how information, decision support, and expert systems represent and enable the evolution of data to information to knowledge to wisdom (Figure 4). For some additional details on an emerging wisdom model, see Appendix A.

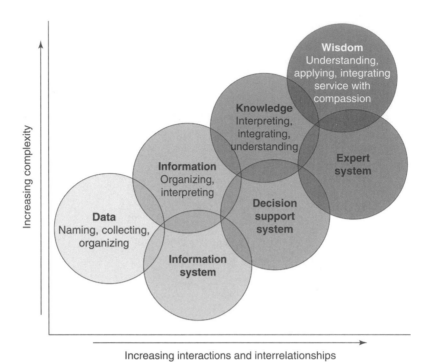

Figure 4. Moving from Data to Expert Systems Version

Benner (1984) defined the experiential stages of the nursing professional in *Novice to Expert: Excellence and Power in Clinical Nursing Practice.* Englebardt and Nelson (2002) also integrated wisdom into their model. Benner, Hooper-Kyriakidis, and Stannard (2011) have contributed Thinking-in-Action as an approach to administration of care. The addition of wisdom raises new and important research questions, challenging the profession to develop tools and processes for classifying, measuring, and encoding wisdom as it relates to nursing and informatics education. Research in these directions will help clarify the relationship between wisdom and the intuitive thinking of expert nurses. Such research will also be invaluable in building information systems to better support healthcare practitioners in decision-making.

Integration of Nursing Informatics into Practice

Data, information, knowledge, and wisdom are central to effective healthcare delivery. Nurses are skilled in managing and communicating information and are always concerned with content quality. Nursing informatics is also concerned with the creation, structure, storage, delivery, exchange, interoperability, and reuse of nursing and clinical information along the continuum of care. As electronic health information systems are integrated into every nursing role and setting, the use of technology at the point of care delivery; the external use of clinical information for quality, legal, and regulatory activities; and the use of analytics of data and metadata contribute to the creation of new nursing knowledge. Such an evolution in the healthcare environment and ubiquitous use of data, information, and knowledge resources contribute to the blurring of the boundaries between the roles of nurses, informatics nurses, and informatics nurse specialists.

The *informatics nurse (IN)* is a registered nurse with an interest or experience in an informatics field, most often identified as nursing informatics. The informatics nurse specialist (INS) is a registered nurse with formal graduate-level education in informatics or an informatics-related field. The informatics nurse specialist is often responsible for implementing or coordinating projects involving multiple professions and specialties. Both INs and INSs employ their unique informatics knowledge, experience, and skills to support and enable other registered nurses to best use data, information, knowledge, and technology in their practice domain. They interact with healthcare consumers and other diverse stakeholders across all care settings and throughout the entire system life cycle.

Nursing Informatics Practice

As previously presented, *nursing informatics (NI)* is the specialty that integrates nursing science with multiple information and analytical sciences to identify, define, manage, and communicate data, information, knowledge, and wisdom in nursing practice. NI supports nurses, consumers, patients, the interprofessional healthcare team, and other stakeholders in their decision-making in all roles and settings to achieve desired outcomes. This support is accomplished through the use of information structures, information processes, and information technology.

Note that information technology does not define NI. The synthesis of data and information into knowledge and wisdom is a core principle of NI, while information technology supports a system lifecycle process. Both the IN and the INS strive to master information management and information technology in the design, structure, retrieval, presentation, storage, exchange, and use of data, information, and knowledge. The IN and INS consider the impact of information and applied computer science on healthcare delivery and the nursing process. Table 1 illustrates the connection between the different foci of nursing and NI. These occur along a continuum without distinct boundaries.

Table 1. Nursing and Nursing Informatics Foci	
Nursing Focus	**Nursing Informatics Focus**
Nurses, patients, health, environment	Information user, information recipients, exchange of data, information, knowledge, and wisdom
Content of information, support for evidence-based practice	Design, structure, interpretation, and representation of data, information, knowledge, and wisdom
Using information applications and technology	Design, develop, implement, and evaluate applications and technologies, ensuring their safety, quality, effectiveness, efficiency, and usability

Tenets of Nursing Informatics

The following tenets of nursing informatics form a framework that characterizes the thinking and actions of informatics nurses in all aspects of practice and in every setting. Nursing informatics

- Has a unique body of knowledge, preparation, and experience that aligns with the nursing profession. NI incorporates informatics concepts in specific application to the role of nursing and nurses in the healthcare continuum.

- Involves the synthesis of data and information into knowledge and wisdom.

- Supports the decision-making of healthcare consumers, nurses, and other professionals in all roles and settings to achieve healthcare consumer safety and advocacy.

- Supports data analytics, including quality-of-care measures, to improve population health outcomes and global health. The IN and INS understand that the real-time application of accurate information by nurses and other clinicians is a mechanism to change healthcare delivery and affect patient outcomes.

- Promotes data integrity and the access and exchange of health data for all consumers of health information.

- Supports national and international agendas on interoperability and the efficient and effective transfer and delivery of data, information, and knowledge.

- Ensures that collaboration is an integral characteristic of practice.

- Interleaves user experience and computer–human interaction concepts throughout practice.

- Incorporates key ethical concerns of NI such as advocacy, privacy, and assurance of the confidentiality and security of data and information.

- Considers the impact of technological changes on patient safety, health-care delivery, quality reporting, and the nursing process.

- Leads in the design and promotion of useful, innovative information technologies that advance practice and achieve desired outcomes.

Nursing, the Nursing Process, and Vocabularies

"Nursing is the protection, promotion, and optimization of health and abilities, prevention of illness and injury, alleviation of suffering through the diagnosis and treatment of human response, and advocacy in the care of individuals, families, communities, and populations" (ANA, 2010). Further explication of nursing practice and its complexity is found in the established standards of professional nursing practice that incorporate the nursing process of assessment, diagnosis, outcomes identification, planning, implementation, and evaluation. Delineated competencies accompany each standard.

The importance of languages, vocabularies, and terminologies cannot be overstated when describing nursing practice. Nursing leaders have identified many different vocabularies and ways of organizing data, information, and knowledge pertinent to nursing through numerous established research initiatives that have spanned decades. In the early 1990s, ANA began to formally recognize these languages, vocabularies, and terminologies (listed in Table 2) as valuable representations of nursing practice and to promote the integration of standardized terminologies into information technology solutions. To date, none has emerged as the leading standardized resource able to represent all nursing practice concepts.

Table 2. ANA Recognized Terminologies and Data Element Sets		
ANA-Recognized Informatics Systems	**Setting Where Developed**	**Content**
Data Element Sets		
NMDS Nursing Minimum Data Set	All nursing	Clinical data elements
NMMDS Nursing Management Minimum Data Set	All settings	Nursing administrative data elements
Nursing-Developed Terminologies		
CCC System Clinical Care Classification System	All nursing care + other health professionals	Diagnoses, interventions, and outcomes
ICNP® International Classification for Nursing Practice	All nursing	Diagnoses, interventions, and outcomes
NANDA NANDA International	All nursing	Diagnoses
NIC Nursing Interventions Classification	All nursing	Interventions
NOC Nursing Outcomes Classification	All nursing	Outcomes
Omaha System	Home care, public health, and community	Diagnoses, interventions, and outcomes
PNDS Perioperative Nursing Data Set	Perioperative care settings	Diagnoses, interventions, and outcomes
Multidisciplinary Terminologies		
ABC ABC Codes	Nursing and other health professionals	Interventions
LOINC® Logical Observation Identifiers, Names, and Codes	Nursing and other health professionals	Outcomes and assessments
SNOMED CT Systematic Nomenclature of Medicine Clinical Terms	Nursing and other health professionals	Diagnoses, interventions, and outcomes

Adapted from ANA, 2012.

Standardized terminologies have become a significant vehicle for facilitating interoperability between different concepts, nomenclatures, and information systems. Continued evolution, mapping, and integration of concepts, as well as research efforts, characterize today's terminology environment in light of passage of the Health Information Technology for Economic and Clinical Health (HITECH) Act of 2009. HITECH's accompanying funding resources continue to stimulate more rapid movement toward electronic data capture and health information exchanges (HIEs) (HealthIT.gov, 2009). Two examples follow.

> *The International Classification for Nursing Practice (ICNP®), developed and maintained by the International Council of Nurses (ICN), provides a global cross-map of nursing terminologies to unite nursing practice through comparison, new research generation, and to inform and influence health policy. ICNP® has been harmonized with SNOMED CT® and offers more than 18 different translations (ICN, 2013).*

> *The Systematized Nomenclature of Medicine, or SNOMED CT® (http://www.ihtsdo.org/snomed-ct/), is a comprehensive universal healthcare reference terminology and messaging structure. SNOMED CT® enables multiple nursing terminology systems to be mapped to one another through harmonized concepts. Released in 2011, the Nursing Problem List Subset of SNOMED CT® is the primary coding terminology for nursing problems used in clinical documentation and based on nursing concepts found within the National Library of Medicine's Unified Medical Language System (UMLS) Metathesaurus. The UMLS Metathesaurus includes more than 100 source vocabularies and is responsible for managing the nursing terminologies mapped to SNOMED CT®. Other mapping initiatives are underway.*

The U.S. federal government formalized its interest in standardized terms to describe healthcare practice when the Office of the National Coordinator for Health Information Technology (ONC) established the HIT Standards Committee with its role to recommend the clinical vocabularies to be used in the electronic specification process (Table 3). Clinical vocabularies define the concepts used to measure clinical processes and patient outcomes. Harmonization between the different vocabularies is necessary to ensure appropriate implementation of the electronic measures across all electronic health record (EHR) systems. This table does not

Table 3. ONC HIT Standards Committee Recommended Clinical Vocabulary Standards		
Vocabulary	**Setting Application**	**Content**
CVX Codes for Vaccines Administered	Nursing and other	Vaccines (administered)
CPT Current Procedural Terminology	Other	Medical, surgical, and diagnostic services rendered for claims
CDC-PHIN/VADS CDC-Public Health Information Network/Vocabulary Access and Distribution System	Nursing and other	Patient characteristic (administrative gender, date of birth)
HCPCS Healthcare Common Procedure Coding System	Other	Medical, surgical, and diagnostic services rendered for claims
ICD-9 CM International Statistical Classification of Diseases and Related Health Problems—Clinical Modification (9th ed.)	Nursing and other	Diagnoses and assessments
ICD-9 PCS International Statistical Classification of Diseases and Related Health Problems— Procedural Coding System (9th ed.)	Nursing and other	Diagnoses and assessments
ICD-10 CM International Statistical Classification of Diseases and Related Health Problems—Clinical Modification (10th ed.)	Nursing and other	Diagnoses and assessments
ICD-10 PCS International Statistical Classification of Diseases and Related Health Problems—Procedural Coding System (10th ed.)	Nursing and other	Diagnoses and assessments
ICF International Classification of Functioning, Disability, and Health	Nursing and other	Functional status

ISO-639 International Organization for Standardization Standard 639	Nursing and other	Representation of languages and language groups
LOINC® Logical Observation Identifiers, Names, and Codes	Nursing and other	Outcomes and assessments
RxNORM	Nursing and other	Normalized clinical drug names
SNOMED CT® Systematic Nomenclature of Medicine Clinical Terms	Nursing and other	Diagnoses, interven- tions, and outcomes
UCUM Unified Code for Units of Measure	Nursing and other	Units of measure for results

Adapted from CMS Measures Management System Blueprint v. 11.0, July 2014
(http://www.cms.gov/Medicare/Quality-Initiatives-Patient-Assessment-Instruments/
MMS/MeasuresManagementSystemBlueprint.html).

include recognition of the important codes reflected in the *Fifth Edition of the Diagnostic and Statistical Manual of Mental Disorders (DSM-5)* released in 2013.

Such diversity and disparity confirm that informatics nurses must seek a broader picture of the implications of their work and the uses of languages and vocabularies for documentation by end users and in outcomes analysis. For instance, nurses mapping a home care vocabulary to an intervention vocabulary must see beyond the technical aspect of the work to understand how a case manager for a multisystem health organization or a home care agency may be basing knowledge of nursing acuity and case mix on the differing vocabularies. By envisioning the varied uses of the terminologies, the IN and INS promote continuity in the patient care process by harmonizing concepts across disparate organizations and EHR systems. Success in this area mandates active informatics nurse participation in associated standards initiatives, such as the work being done by Health Level Seven International (HL7) and the International Health Terminology Standards Development Organisation (IHTSDO).

Concepts and Tools from Information Science and Computer Science

Tools and methods from information and computer sciences are fundamental to NI, including:

- Information management—An elemental process by which one files, stores, manipulates, and reports data for various uses.

- Information communication—Enables systems to send data and to present information in formats that improve understanding.

- Information structures—Organize data, information, and knowledge for processing by computers.

- Information technology—Includes computer hardware, software, communication, and network technologies, derived primarily from computer science. Its use distinguishes informatics from more traditional methods of information management.

User Experience and Related Concepts

Usability, human–computer interaction (HCI), ergonomics, and human factors have long been overlapping concepts of fundamental interest to the informatics nurse. Contemporary thinking has identified *user experience* as the overarching descriptive term.

Although the 2001 Institute of Medicine (IOM) report, *Crossing the Quality Chasm: A New Health System for the 21st Century,* publicized the importance of human factors in health care, the emphasis for attention and action related to usability goes much further. Many researchers (including Ash, Berg, & Coiera, 2004; Ash, Sittig, Dykstra, Campbell, & Guappone, 2009; Koppel et al., 2005; Staggers, Jennings, & Lasome, 2010; and Guo, Irdbarren, Kapsandoy, Perri, & Staggers, 2011) have reported usability issues. Stead and Lin (2009) concluded from their evaluation of top U.S. electronic health records that the major impediment to their effectiveness was usability.

ISO 9241-11 defines *usability* as the extent to which a product can be used by specific users in a specific context to achieve specific goals with effectiveness, efficiency, and satisfaction. Usability in healthcare is fundamentally about patient safety and human performance with tools and systems. Several resources provide more details about usability:

- Health Information and Management Systems Society (HIMSS), *Promoting Usability in Health Organizations: Initial Steps and*

Progress Toward a Healthcare Usability Maturity Model (2011), available at http://www.himss.org/files/HIMSSorg/content/files/ HIMSS_Promoting_Usability_in_Health_Org.pdf

■ National Institute of Standards and Technology (NIST), "Usability" web page, available at http://www.nist.gov/healthcare/usability/

■ U.S. Food and Drug Administration (FDA), "General Human Factors Information and Resource" web page, available at http://www.fda. gov/medicaldevices/deviceregulationandguidance/humanfactors/ ucm124829.htm

■ Tiger Initiative, *Designing Usable Clinical Information Systems: Recommendations from the TIGER Usability and Clinical Application Design Collaborative Team*, available at http://www.thetigerinitiative. org/docs/TigerReport_Usability 000.pdf

■ Jakob Nielsen of the Nielsen Norman Group (2012), "Usability 101: Introduction to Usability," available at http://www.nngroup.com/articles/ usability-101-introduction-to-usability/

HCI examines how people, software applications, and computer technology interact and influence each other. Elements of HCI are rooted in psychology, cognitive science, sociology, computer science, and information science. HCI addresses the design, development, procurement, implementation, and evaluation of applications as well as other components associated with the system life cycle. For example, an informatics nurse would assess a bar-code medication administration system before purchase to determine whether the design and operation complement the way nurses cognitively process medication administration and document that action.

The IOM's 2012 report, *Health IT and Patient Safety: Building Safer Systems for Better Care*, identifies the importance of HCI in the integration of applications and technology with healthcare delivery. Such integration into everyday life has contributed to the empowerment of patients, now often designated as *e-patients*, and the promotion of interprofessional collaboration through mobile technology (m-health). This requires the IN and INS to address all environments and all levels of user ability to assure accommodation of the various devices being developed.

The IN and INS will also have to consider a variety of sociotechnical issues and their effect on HCI (Sittig & Singh, 2010). These include clinical experience level (Cho, Staggers, & Park, 2010), user literacy and user physical limitations

(Huang, Chen, & Chung, 2005), and aging (Sibley, 2008). In the future, the convenience of technologies available in commercial products can be expected to drive similar functionality in healthcare technology and will increase the scope of HCI factors. Finally, the effect of natural language processing (Zhou, 2007) and implantable monitoring devices (Topol, 2011) on HCI is yet to be determined.

The term *ergonomics* refers to attributes of physical equipment or to principles of arrangement of equipment in the work environment. For instance, an informatics nurse may have a role in ensuring that sound ergonomics principles are used in clinical settings to guide the selection and arrangement of various devices to support workflow for interprofessional providers, patients and their families, and other end users.

In the past, HCI, usability, and ergonomics have typically been subsumed under the rubric of *human factors*, or how humans interact with tools, including technology. The Human Factors and Ergonomics Society (HFES) identifies *ergonomics* (or human factors) as "the scientific discipline concerned with the understanding of interactions among humans and other elements of a system, and the profession that applies theory, principles, data and methods to design in order to optimize human well-being and overall system performance" (https://www.hfes.org/web/educationalresources/hfedefinitionsmain. html#profsoc). The concepts of efficiency, effectiveness, and safety are integral and apply to the client, consumer, and others.

The term *user experience* encompasses all aspects of users' interactions. The International Organization for Standardization (ISO) 9241-11 defines the term as "a person's perceptions and responses that result from the use or anticipated use of a product, system or service." (ISO, 2009) describes it as a range of experiences, from walking into a healthcare facility to designs that fit into complex ecosystems with many users interacting. Development of high-quality user experiences requires the diverse expertise of many professions, such as engineering, graphic and industrial design, interface design, and psychology. Staggers (2014) identified the interrelationship of the user experience as encompassing human factors, HCI, ergonomics, and usability, as displayed in Figure 5.

Phenomenon of Nursing

The metaparadigm of nursing comprises four key concepts: nurse, person, health, and environment. The phenomenon of nursing, both art and science, is supported by the tenets of nursing informatics. The nurse continuously collects data about persons, their health, and the environmental factors that

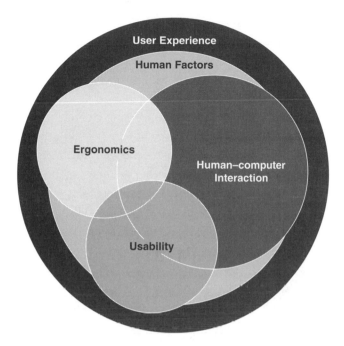

Figure 5. Relationship of User Experience to Other Concepts
Reference: Staggers, 2014, p. 337.

influence health maintenance and the healing process. Nurses, using their education, intellect, and experiential knowledge, place these data into categories to create information. Finally, using critical thinking and wisdom, the nurse is able to formulate a plan and prioritize interventions or actions that effect the most positive outcome possible for the situation.

Nurses make decisions from their unique perspectives based on their education, experience, and specialty. *Decision-making* is the process of choosing among alternatives. The decisions that nurses make can be characterized both by the quality of decisions and by the impact of the actions resulting from those decisions. As knowledge workers, nurses make numerous decisions that affect the lives and well-being of individuals, families, groups, communities, and populations. The process of decision-making in nursing is guided by the concept of critical thinking. *Critical thinking* is the intellectually disciplined process of actively and skillfully searching out the best evidence and using that knowledge to conceptualize, apply, analyze, synthesize, and/or evaluate data and information as a guide to belief and action (adapted from Scriven & Paul, 1987).

The nursing process of assessment, diagnosis, outcomes identification, planning, implementation, and evaluation can be enhanced through the utilization of technology. Technology, when properly developed and applied, has been shown to enhance the healthcare team's ability to collect, categorize, interpret, manage, evaluate, and share relevant information. This also enhances the team's ability to manage client care in a more efficient and productive manner. In most cases, the utilization of technology has decreased the nurse's workload associated with collecting and categorizing data, while enabling and enhancing the sharing of relevant information with other members of the healthcare team. When the complexity of information sharing is decreased, enhanced sharing of relevant information within the healthcare team theoretically improves quality and safety and results in improved patient outcomes. The informatics nurse is ideally suited to evaluate how technology can assist the nurse and other members of the care delivery team to manage data and share information to achieve desired outcomes.

In addition to enhancing the nursing process, data collection, information sharing, intervention implementation, and resultant patient outcomes can be tracked via database queries and processed through research methods. Evidence-based practice models can be developed through this research. Models of practice that generate positive patient outcomes can then be replicated and supported by systems optimized to allow seamless data capture, intuitive data display, and expert system processing.

Nursing is focused on optimizing the health status of individuals, families, groups, communities, and populations. Each of these entities is affected by the environment in which it resides. Technology, when properly designed and implemented, enhances the ability to track and trend data to help determine what, where, when, how, and why resources could be allocated to achieve the greatest good. Informatics nurses are uniquely qualified to assist in the development and optimization of systems that capture, categorize, share, and evaluate data and information while keeping the nursing process as the foundation of practice.

Functional Areas of Nursing Informatics

Informatics nurses, informatics nurse specialists, and other stakeholders are helping transform health care through the use of informatics processes, tools, and structures. Across all healthcare environments, INs and INSs most commonly practice in interprofessional healthcare environments and interact with information technology (IT) professionals during all phases of the system life cycle. INs and INSs use scientific and informatics principles and employ creative strategies in informatics solutions. They bring the perspectives of nursing, and very often the patients, to interprofessional work through a solid understanding of operational processes and the value of consumer advocacy to informatics functions. INs and INSs may need additional education or other types of advanced preparation to manage the informatics projects at hand.

Because of the tendency to confuse roles with titles, this section describes the following dynamic and evolving functional areas of nursing informatics:

- Administration, leadership, and management

- Systems analysis and design

- Compliance and integrity management

- Consultation

- Coordination, facilitation, and integration

- Development of systems, products, and resources

- Educational and professional development

- Genetics and genomics

- Information management/operational architecture

- Policy development and advocacy

- Quality and performance improvement

- Research and evaluation

- Safety, security, and environmental health

The last discussion in this section describes additional integrated functions, especially those crossing clinical practice and informatics. INs and INSs may be in positions that focus primarily on one functional area; more frequently, though, several functional areas are combined within a particular NI position.

Administration, Leadership, and Management

As is true of administration in general, leadership and management functions in nursing informatics incorporate both higher-level and mid-level administrative functions. Increasingly, INSs are attaining senior leadership positions. Positions may be titled Chief Nursing Informatics Officer (CNIO), Chief Information

Officer (CIO), director, or similar leadership titles (American Organization of Nurse Executives [AONE], 2012; Hodges & Wierz, 2012). In this functional capacity, nursing informatics leaders are expected to be visionary and establish the direction of large-scale informatics solutions. The nursing informatics leader often serves as a catalyst for developing strategic plans and creating national or system policies and procedures, while serving as the champion for integrated projects and systems.

In mid-level management, INSs may supervise resources and activities for all phases of the system life cycle. These activities may include needs analysis, requirements gathering, design, development, selection and purchase, testing, implementation, and evaluation of systems to support all facets of nursing and healthcare delivery. At all levels, leadership is characterized by the combination of superb communication skills, collaboration, change management, risk assessment, and coalition building with political finesse, business acumen, and strategic application knowledge. INSs serving in this functional area may put most of their energy into leadership and management. In other positions, administration may be part of a position merged with other functional areas. Typical examples include:

- INS at a large hospital system, supervising an implementation and education team, representing nursing interests on various IT committees, performing project management for multiple documentation projects, and having oversight of nursing standards and vocabularies used in applications.

- Project director for a clinical software company, managing implementation teams for various client projects (hospitals to ambulatory facilities) and consulting with clients on all aspects of systems selection, customization, adoption, and use of software.

- Grants administrator for an information science research agency, seeking and writing grants that would fund NI-related projects, designing budgets, and ensuring optimal allocation of resources.

A crucial responsibility for any nursing informatics leader is fostering interprofessional collaboration in designing, developing, and deploying technology in healthcare settings. Interprofessional collaborative practice has been defined as occurring "when multiple health workers from different professional backgrounds work together with patients, families, carers [sic], and communities to deliver the highest quality of care" (World Health Organization [WHO], 2010, p. 13). Although informatics nurses may lead teams and projects, the output of these teams rarely has an impact only on nursing care. Most commonly these efforts reflect concerns and actions of interprofessional stakeholders. The Interprofessional Education Collaborative Expert Panel (2011, p. 14) described multiple core competencies for interprofessional teamwork that included "21st-century technologies for communication and coordination (i.e., informatics)," emphasizing how vital it is for all informatics nurse leaders to work collaboratively with all members of the healthcare team.

Systems Analysis and Design

Data can be aggregated and analyzed in a number of ways to synthesize knowledge, inform decision support and outcomes management, advance the science of nursing informatics, and support reimbursement. The IN and INS may use a number of tools and resources to accomplish these ends, such as data flow diagrams, entity-relationship modeling, taxonomies, clinical vocabularies, and quality indicators. Meta-analysis can identify large-scale trends across multiple groups of data. Systems requirements analysis can track the flow of data in a process or system to aid in customization for end-user needs.

A major responsibility of the IN or INS is to understand workflow processes, particular informatics solutions, and how these affect each other. Workflow analysis (identifying the individual tasks of a work process), coupled with an understanding of the clinical process, is essential to enhance safety and reduce inefficiencies in a healthcare environment. Processes must be designed for successful interactions between users and computers. Competence in formal systems analysis techniques permits comparison of systems' capabilities and limitations and is required to design (or redesign) applications for successful computer–user interactions or user experiences.

INs and INSs may also engage in the process of knowledge discovery in databases (KDD). Using sound methodologies and practical evidence-based recommendations, the INS can discover information and knowledge related to diverse areas of nursing practice. Knowledge discovery methods (data mining and machine learning methods) in combination with statistical analysis and data visualization techniques help identify and understand patterns in very large data stores, such as enterprise data warehouses.

Analysis is also required for the use of clinical vocabularies, languages, and taxonomies. Nursing languages must be periodically re-evaluated for their applicability and currency. Analysis of a meta-database, such as the Unified Medical Language System (UMLS), requires knowledge of nursing and medical vocabularies in order to analyze groups of taxonomies and map them to similar terms. An example is the effort to map SNOMED CT to the International

Classification of Diseases, Tenth Revision, Clinical Modification (ICD-10-CM) to aid in meeting and attesting to meaningful use requirements. IN and INS expertise should be included in these efforts to support the collection, reporting, and analysis of nursing-sensitive data.

Outcomes analysis may be related to any domain of nursing practice: clinical, education, research, or administration. The complexity and levels of outcomes must be determined for healthcare consumers, populations, and institutions. Analysis can include the use of humancomputer interaction principles and methods. In that domain, INs and INSs use HCI tools and methods, such as heuristics and cognitive walk-through, to evaluate the match of systems to users, tasks, and contexts.

Analysts use other tools to (1) maintain data integrity and reliability, (2) facilitate data aggregation and analysis, (3) identify outcomes, (4) identify organizational barriers, and (5) develop performance measures. These techniques allow nurses to contribute to building a knowledge base consisting of the data, information, theories, and models used by nurses and other stakeholders in decision-making that supports quality health care. The following are examples of analysis activities:

- A nursing analyst in a hospice setting tracks health consumer data to establish a weighted case mix to determine nursing personnel allocations.

- A quality improvement (QI) specialist in a hospital system aggregates multisite research data related to diagnosis and nursing procedures or risk mapping.

- A quality assurance (QA) analyst works with nurse managers to retool current work processes after examining existing system data in customized QA reports.

- An analyst applies knowledge discovery methods to warehoused electronic data to build a predictive model of patient falls.

- A behavior analyst identifies organizational barriers or breakdowns to avoid system failures or risk.

Compliance and Integrity Management

Following the report *To Err Is Human: Building a Safer Health System* (IOM, 1999), the downfall of Enron, passage of the Sarbanes-Oxley Act of 2002 (SOX), and pay-for-performance incentives adopted by the Centers for Medicare & Medicaid Services (CMS), healthcare organizations must have robust reporting systems to monitor compliance and integrity of their information and reporting activities, infrastructures, employees, and business partners. Along with developing organizational cultures that encourage ethical conduct and regulatory compliance, mechanisms must be in place to prevent and detect criminal conduct.

Computerized information systems must support compliance with the 1996 Health Insurance Portability and Accountability Act (HIPAA) efforts by limiting access to personally identifiable health information to only those who require and are authorized access. Auditing systems that detect red flags, reporting systems that will preserve confidentiality or anonymity, and enterprise risk management (ERM) allow reporting of risks by everyone in an organization. ERM breaks down silos and provides timely reporting of risks and opportunities at a high level for immediate attention through risk scoring and mapping (Carroll & Nakamura, 2011).

The IN and INS must have and maintain the knowledge to effectively apply current ethical standards and regulatory requirements to help healthcare organizations to:

- Revise operational procedures for staff.

- Establish technical processes to maintain compliance.

- Meet new regulatory mandates at local, state, national, and global levels.

These standards, directives, guidelines, or mandates may include those from government agencies, such as the Centers for Medicare & Medicaid Services, the Food and Drug Administration (FDA), the Centers for Disease Control and Prevention (CDC), the National Institutes of Health (NIH), and accreditation organizations, such as The Joint Commission (TJC), Healthcare Facilities Accreditation Program (HFAP), Det Norske Veritas Healthcare, Inc. (DNV), and the World Health Organization (WHO).

Ethical issues surround the use of new products, such as embedded technologies and radio-frequency identification (RFID), which can be used in caring for persons with Alzheimer's disease and other dementias. As the science matures, some of these issues will be resolved and standards will be established. Requirements will continue to evolve. The following are examples of compliance and integrity management activities:

- The security officer for a hospital ensures that HIPAA standards are met by software vendors within the organization, periodically monitors software audit logs for breaches, and ensures that passwords are not shared and that backup and disaster procedures are in place and operational.

- A compliance officer for a state health agency writes and enforces policies that conform to state and national laws respecting records retention.

- A care coordinator administrator for a hospital system ensures the confidentiality of data transmitted via telehealth and telemedicine devices.

- An internal auditor reviews charges to documented care given for appropriate reimbursement or abnormal billing practices.

Consultation

Informatics nurses and informatics nurse specialists apply informatics knowledge and skills to serve as transformational leaders and resources for clients, both formally and informally, in external and internal settings. Informatics nurse consultants are expected to have solid expertise in clinical nursing and areas such as process redesign, strategic IT planning, system implementation, writing for informatics and other publications, evaluating clinical software products, working with clients to write requests for proposals, performing market research, and assisting in the planning of conferences, academic courses, and professional development programs. Expert INSs may serve as internal consultants, work for a consulting firm, own an independent practice, and be recognized as experts by writing about NI and speaking at NI-related events. Flexibility, good communication skills, solid nursing/healthcare delivery background, breadth and depth of clinical and informatics knowledge, and excellent interpersonal skills are needed to respond to rapidly changing projects and priorities. Project examples include:

- Consulting with individuals and groups in defining healthcare information problems and identifying methods for implementing, utilizing, and modifying IT solutions and data structures to support healthcare access, delivery, and evaluation.

- Consulting as the project manager to identify strengths, weaknesses, opportunities, and threats; to ensure that team members are performing duties as assigned; and to complete the project on time and within budget.

- Consulting with clients in writing requests for proposals to elicit vendor bids for informatics solutions and in evaluating vendor responses.

Coordination, Facilitation, and Integration

One of the most common NI roles is implementing informatics solutions. Nurses are particularly well suited for IT implementation, as it essentially follows the nursing process of assessment, diagnosis, outcomes identification, planning, implementation, and evaluation (ANA, 2010). The IN or INS may serve as project coordinator, facilitating change management and integrating the information and technology to transform processes. In this role, project management knowledge and skills are essential to the success of the project. Project coordination can range from small, department-centered efforts to enterprise-wide initiatives. Examples include:

■ Coordinating installations, system upgrades, and optimization of existing features and functions.

■ Employing research methodologies to disseminate new knowledge and integrate that knowledge into practice.

■ Developing and defining healthcare policy to advance public health.

■ Serving as a systems administrator of a learning management system (LMS) for the delivery of e-learning courses or training programs for healthcare professionals.

The IN and INS frequently serve as a hub for interprofessional communication and as a bridge and communication liaison between and among informatics solution users, clinical and nonclinical end users, and IT experts and staff. The IN and INS often serve as translators and integrators addressing system requirements and impacts.

Informatics nurses frequently serve as the liaison between engineers and end users. In this capacity, the informatics nurse ensures that necessary testing or research is performed to determine the end user's needs and that information is conveyed appropriately. The informatics nurse will also play a key role in the development and testing of new applications or enhancements to existing applications. Once the engineer has created a product, the informatics nurse evaluates the use and usability of the product from the viewpoint of the end user. This liaison type of facilitation and coordination occurs in multiple environments. Ensuring the integration of nursing vocabularies and standardized nomenclatures in applications is another example. In this case INs and INSs can also act as usability experts and recommend ideal formats for the utilization of technology. Examples of coordination, facilitation, and integration include:

■ The project coordinator for a statewide electronic health record implementation coordinates all aspects of the project and supervises an interdisciplinary team to prepare public health personnel to use the application.

■ The project manager for a clinical software company (using tools such as project management software and project plans) manages the resources and activities for clients whose responsibilities cross inpatient and ambulatory areas.

■ The clinical liaison for a telehealth software vendor communicates with providers and consumers to ensure that all parties are agreeable to development and implementation plans, and ensures that providers using the system receive adequate technical education.

■ A usability expert on a software development team advises software engineers on screen design from the standpoint of clinical documentation needs, performs or coordinates testing of iterative designs, and validates clinical requirements with the users.

Development of Systems, Products, and Resources

A developer is responsible for translating user requirements into effective informatics solutions. Informatics nurses are involved in a vast array of development activities, from conceptualizing models for applications, to software and hardware design, to the design of education manuals and media, to the design of complex technology networks. As part of this function, INs and INSs participate in the process of design, iterative development, testing, and dissemination of quality informatics solutions for nurses, other healthcare professionals, and consumers. An understanding of the information needs of nurses and the nursing profession, consumers and consumer care processes, best business practices, client services, projected market directions, product design and development methods, market research, contemporary programming, systems design, and modeling language are essential for practicing in a development environment.

Adherence to national standards and regulatory requirements is also essential to any development work. To ensure interoperability between systems, INs and INSs involved in system development must be knowledgeable about international standards requirements. Existing standards include Health Level Seven (HL7), International Organization for Standardization (ISO), Current Procedural Terminology (CPT), International Statistical Classification of Disease and Related Health Problems (ICD), and Digital Imaging and Communications in Medicine (DICOM) group standards, as well as Section 508 accessibility standards. An understanding of the current work on standards is mandatory. The following are examples of development responsibilities:

- A developer employed by a personal health record software vendor creates user-friendly screens for consumers to enter information as well as screens for nurses to display and interpret the data.

- A database administrator with a large multisite teaching organization manages an expanded nursing vocabulary set for inpatient, ambulatory, and home health nursing documentation.

- A nurse Web content developer for a consortium creates and validates content for educational handouts, help and tool tips for user interfaces that display national guidelines, and educational tools. This content includes new and innovative tools for knowledge dissemination.

- A programmer in a hospital IT department codes software for documenting diabetic education.

Education and Professional Development

Education is a critical component of many NI functions and may directly affect the success or failure of any new or modified IT solution. Vendors of information systems frequently use the term *training* when referring to client education. In nursing, however, the broader label of *education* is used. Adherence to solid educational principles is a necessary component of education and professional development. Teaching nurses and nursing students, healthcare consumers and families, and members of the interprofessional healthcare team about the effective and ethical uses of information technology, as well as NI concepts and theories, is essential for the optimal use of informatics solutions in nursing practice. Ever-changing requirements in health information technology make continuing education essential as well. INs and INSs in this capacity develop, implement, and evaluate educational curricula and educational technologies to meet learners' needs.

In this role, educators and trainers assess and evaluate informatics skills and competencies while providing feedback to the learner regarding the effectiveness of the activity and the learner's ability to demonstrate newly acquired skills. Educators and trainers manage, evaluate, report, and utilize data and information related to the specific learner and the educational delivery system. These informatics nurse innovators define and develop educational technologies, integrate the solutions into the educational and practice environments, and challenge organizations to consider and adopt innovative informatics solutions. The introduction of mobile technologies provides an opportunity for additional creative learning methodologies.

The informatics nurse must evaluate the users' level of information literacy as well as their computer literacy. Computer literacy is a core competency needed in health care and nursing practice, and should be taught in nursing curricula at all levels. In addition, information literacy must be integrated into practice and used to support knowledge management. These are the foundations of informatics competencies.

Education and professional development must include INs, INSs, end users, and consumers. The use of innovative technologies to support telehealth/telemonitoring and mobile health (mHealth) has encouraged the use of Internet-based consumer-accessible applications, especially by older adults. New competencies are needed to ensure that health information is displayed to consumers at an appropriate level of understanding for all delivery devices, so that support staff personnel are rarely needed. Cultural issues, language considerations, and literacy levels must be assessed and accommodated prior to implementation.

Informatics nurses need to ensure that the content of web-based knowledge portals of both private and government health organizations are reliable, accurate, and trustworthy. Education and professional development involve not only education of INs and INSs, but also development of appropriate user interfaces for the consumer and other healthcare team members. Examples of education and professional development functions include:

- An academic role teaching the basic NI principles to all levels of nursing students or preparing graduate nursing students enrolled in a nursing informatics degree program to implement, support, and evaluate clinical applications.

- A development role creating simulation technology scenarios and curricula to support traditional learning and clinical placements.

- A clinical preceptor role orienting newly hired nurses and students to the use of telehealth, telehealth technology, and mHealth technologies, integrating these technologies into clinical practice, and then providing consumer education.

- A vendor educator role involving international travel to educate nurses on the operations, capabilities, troubleshooting, limitations, and benefits of a product.

- A staff development liaison role for a large hospital educating nurses and other end users about how to integrate clinical applications into their work processes.

■ A consultant role assisting a clinician practice with the implementation, use, and ongoing support of electronic health records and other related technologies.

■ Working as a help desk team member assisting users with support during clinical application upgrades/releases, answering clinical user questions, or trouble-shooting user problems.

■ A patient education coordinator role facilitating electronic consumer health resources.

■ Web developer responsibilities for development, maintenance, and presentation of disease content for a hospital web portal.

■ Oversight of social media resources, products, and policies to enhance this evolving and important communication technology, enabling open and enhanced communication among healthcare consumers, providers, vendors, and other stakeholders.

Genetics and Genomics

Advances in mapping the human genome and understanding the character-istics and influence of individual DNA have had a dramatic impact on what is known about patients. These data, especially when integrated into EHRs or personal health records (PHRs), are leading to innovations in patient care and customized medications and therapies targeted to the individual's unique responses. Care and medication can be more precisely individualized to patients based on their unique DNA profiles. Data about their past response to medica-tions and other interventions can be documented. This is dramatically chang-ing how patients are being managed for specific diseases and conditions and is extending into the prevention of some diseases.

Computerized clinical decision support can help manage the inherent complexity of customized patient care. Predictive disease models based on patients' DNA profiles are emerging as clinicians better understand DNA mapping. These advances have significant implications for a new model of care and for the IN's and INS's participation in the development of genomic IT solutions. More than ever, patients will need to be partners in this develop-ment. Genomics is leading to many specialized advances in care delivery and must be linked to exact, individualized data within a personal health record. Subsequently, advanced disease management with the ultimate goal of disease prevention will be possible. This change has many implications for ethics as well as informatics. In fact, genomics competencies and curricular guidelines are available online (ANA & ISONG, 2011; http://www.genome.gov/Pages/Health/HealthCareProvidersInfo/Grad_Gen_Comp.pdf).

With the increased amount of research regarding the impact of genomic variation on health and its increasing relevance to clinical practice, informatics nurses need to build their genetics/genomics knowledge base so that they may support this expanding practice area. This involves developing an understanding of genomic bioinformatics, the types of genomic information available, and how such information can be stored and abstracted within the EHR for genomic clinical decision support.

The Genomic Nursing State of the Science Advisory Panel (Calzone et al., 2013) calls for informatics nurses to contribute to the infrastructure for informatics support systems that use genomic information. The genomic nursing science blueprint has specifically targeted innovation supported through nursing research and technology development as a priority, including:

1. "Data storage and use to facilitate research process and outcomes;

2. Facilitate cross-generational sharing of genomic data (e.g., family history, laboratory analyses);

3. Managing, analyzing, and interpreting genomic information (e.g., sequencing data);

4. Point-of-care decision support for client and healthcare provider;

5. Common terminology and taxonomy, and

6. Common formats for data storage/exchange and queries" (Calzone, 2013, p. 100).

Supporting clinical documentation and information system technologies are changing to meet the demands created by the evolution of personalized care and individualized therapies related to an individual's genomic characteristics. Informatics nurses have unique opportunities to engage in requirements definition, design, implementation, and evaluation activities, as well as policy development and ethics discussions.

Information Management and Operational Architecture

Information management (IM) acquires, organizes, controls, disseminates, and uses (reuses) information from any source regardless of origin (internal or external to the organization). Such management efforts address the quality, ownership, use, and security of information in the context of organizational performance to support and achieve the effective operation of an organization (adapted from Feather & Sturges, 2002).

An organization must manage electronic and physical information through the information life cycle, regardless of origin source or format (data, paper documents, electronic documents, wave forms, audio, social media, video, etc.), for delivery through multiple channels (cable, Internet, and broadcast interfaces). Information management includes the capture, management, preservation, storage, and delivery of the right information to the right people at the right time. The informatics nurse's role in information management consists largely of the organization and control of planning, structure, processing, evaluation, and reporting of information activities to meet objectives and enable the delivery of information.

Operational architecture (OpArc) can be used throughout the system life cycle to address the complexity of information exchange through the use of "views" to describe and interrelate the data elements, tasks, activities, and information flows required to accomplish clinical operations. Operational architecture provides a repeatable, standardized, structured, and integrated approach linking operational concepts to the providing healthcare systems, as well as technical standards for the objective analysis of information requirements.

Policy Development and Advocacy

Informatics nurses play a key role in formulation of health policy, in particular bringing expertise in data and information content, data structures, and IT solutions, care coordination, and advocacy. Policy development may be at any level: international, national, regional, state, and local. Informatics nurses are experts in defining the data needed and the structure, management, and availability of those data for decision-making. This allows them to advocate for consumers, providers, and the enterprise, and to articulate relevant issues from a nursing perspective or healthcare consumer viewpoint. Policy-related activities may include developing, writing, implementing, and evaluating guidance. Regardless of the level or activity, informatics nurses are partners in setting health policy, particularly in relation to information management and communication, infrastructure development, and economics.

The advocacy function of the IN or INS also encompasses consumer health. Informatics nurses may be part of initiatives such as promoting the adoption of technology for rural programs to increase access to health services, or endorsing government and private initiatives to engage consumers in creating a personal health record. Advocacy may include educating legislators about such topics as increasing telecommunication access, expanding reimbursement for technology-enabled consumer services, or educating the public on ways to access health-related materials via the Internet. Examples of the policy development and advocacy function of the IN or INS include the following:

- The president of a health information management organization represents nursing on a national information standards task force.

- An informatics nurse lobbyist participates in advocacy efforts on behalf of consumers for increased government funding of demonstration or pilot informatics projects.

- A president of a nursing informatics organization writes letters to elected officials to obtain their support for reimbursement of services by remote, technology-enabled providers.

Quality and Performance Improvement

At present, emphasis is increasingly focused on ensuring seamless integration of quality and performance improvement to enhance patient outcomes. All aspects of healthcare services delivery require access to significant data, information, and knowledge resources. Comparative effectiveness, meaningful use, core quality measures, development of e-clinical measures, and the application of protocols and critical paths will require further development and refinement. The informatics nurse is uniquely positioned to help identify available measurable content and generate queries and reports that trend and track events and actions and respond to specific inquiries, questions, and concerns. This functional role is closely aligned with development, research, evaluation, safety, and security activities described in other sections.

Research and Evaluation

Informatics nurses and informatics nurse specialists may conduct research into the design, development, implementation, and evaluation of informatics solutions, models, and theories. INS researchers use systematic methods of inquiry (including traditional and newer techniques) to identify, retrieve, represent, and evaluate data, information, and knowledge within informatics solutions and data repositories. Research and evaluation functions include, but are not limited to:

- Research in concept or symbolic representation of nursing phenomena.

- Evaluation of clinical decision-making in nursing.

- Applied informatics research.

- Assessment of the use of health information tools and resources by consumers and interprofessional team members.

- Evaluation of effective methods for information systems implementation, acceptance, and utilization.

- User experience research about the design of systems and their impact on interprofessional providers, consumers, nurses, and their interactions.

- Evaluation research about the effects of systems on the processes and outcomes of care and customer satisfaction.

- Usability testing of nursing and consumer applications.

- Evaluating how consumers use computerized healthcare products.

- Research concerning clinical vocabularies.

- Consumer communication and usage of technology-based support groups.

Research in nursing informatics may span a range of activities, including exploratory research (such as data mining), experimental research, process improvement, and informal evaluation. An INS working in research and evaluation might conduct research projects to develop and refine standardized nursing vocabularies, or to link nursing interventions to outcomes in large data sets. This work may include the evaluation of organizational attributes for successful adoption of documentation systems or the impact and efficacy of hardware and software solutions.

Nursing informatics research may also incorporate a consumer orientation, through the study of effective nurse-consumer interactions and communications in web-based interactions with older consumers, or the impact of new applications on nurses' workflow. Patient reactions to instant messaging from providers may be studied. The following are examples of the research function of the INS:

- The chief of nursing research for a large software company oversees projects to evaluate the impact of enterprise electronic health records on patient care outcomes.

■ A nursing informatics analyst in a hospital IT department aggregates data about the incidence of pressure ulcers, creates trend reports and predictive models for nurse managers, and analyzes outcomes against quality indicators.

■ A nurse researcher conducts a usability study comparing consumer entry of information at a clinic-based kiosk to in-person interviews.

Safety, Security, and Environmental Health

The areas of safety and security, as well as environmental health, are rapidly becoming more important concerns for informatics nurses. Informatics nurses have multiple opportunities to assist in assuring the safety and security of health-related IT (HIT) products that support clinicians, as well as patients, families, and other caregivers. Though intended to reduce safety issues, HIT can actually create errors. In 2007, sufficient evidence in the literature gave rise to the term "e-iatrogenesis," denoting harm resulting in part from HIT (Weiner, Kfuri, Chan, & Fowles, 2007). The authors stated that e-iatrogenesis is the most significant unintended consequence of HIT.

The implementation of electronic health records without regard to workflow analysis and redesign, human–computer interaction, prevention of errors in medication administration, and prevention of possible missed diagnoses have increased the concern for patient safety. By 2011, the Institute of Medicine's Committee on Patient Safety and Health Information Technology had released *Health IT and Patient Safety: Building Safer Systems for Better Care*, a 211-page report describing in detail the issues surrounding HIT safety and security. The report included recommendations for software vendors and HIT users on building, integrating, and maintaining safer and more secure systems. It also addressed opportunities for research and policy development. Poor usability is the most significant safety issue currently confronting clinicians. A simple example is the "adjacency error" whereby users mistakenly select an item next to the one intended in a drop-down menu (IOM, 2012).

The increasing deployment and use of HIT to engage patients in their own health care will require a unique strategy to support safety and security. As device and system interoperability expands and "bring your own device" (BYOD) strategies are increasingly deployed to satisfy clinical users and consumers, the associated security and privacy risks, including the susceptibility to malware and hacking, will likewise increase. Additional safety topics that merit attention of informatics nurses include: implementation decisions about prompts and alerts, role-based security for access, authentication, student-instructor signature/authentication, patient access to clinical notes and portals, and impact and opportunities associated with health information exchanges. See the ONC *Health IT Patient Safety Action and Surveillance Plan* (available at http://www.healthit.gov/sites/default/files/safety_plan_master.pdf).

With regard to environmental health and informatics, there are two traditional notions of "environment" in nursing practice: internal and external. In an internal environment, typically some control exists by which the work area can be modified to create safe and comfortable conditions where the nurse cares for, or interacts with, clients. This could be a hospital, clinic, school, or a client's home. An external environment is characterized as offering no, or limited, control in manipulating the climate or environmental hazards. Examples include industrial zones where an occupational health nurse may practice, a neighborhood or public area where a community health nurse may practice, or a disaster zone where a mobile intensive care nurse may be stationed. In both internal and external environments, hazards and/or materials exist that could cause physical or mental injury, such as that resulting from equipment that is not ergonomically designed or correctly grounded. Similarly, hostility and incivility in the work environment must be identified and addressed.

A number of initiatives at the federal (Recordkeeping—The OSHA 300 Log, 2013), state (Agency for Toxic Substances & Disease Registry, 2010), and community (Community Health Nurses' Initiatives Group, 2013) levels actively support the nurse as an integral steward in monitoring and improving environmental safety for healthcare workers and their clients (individuals, families, communities, and populations). In addition, a number of programs are designed to educate nurses in environmental health principles and even achieve certification as a Registered Environmental Health Specialist (Registered Environmental Health Specialist Program, 2013).

Although environmental health is not typically considered part of the informatics nurse's scope of practice, informatics nurses can develop and coordinate education, communication, and reference materials, as well as design system tools that are easily accessible and pertinent to the needs of their colleagues. Some examples of resources are online learning modules, hyperlinks embedded into a clinical documentation tool directing the user to ergonomics information and safety data sheets, and expert system alerts within the clinical documentation system warning the caregiver when the assessment and other criteria show a threat to health and safety of the patient or the nurse, such as radioactive exposure, past violent behavior, or infections.

Creation of a healthy, supportive work environment includes such activities as noise reduction from the hum of electronic equipment and fans and audible alerts and alarms; removal of trip and personal hazards, such as exposed electrical cords and cables, heavy movable but unstable work stations; and exposure to electromagnetic frequencies and potential electric shock. Responsible recycling or disposal of electronic equipment, printer cartridges, and paper printouts reflect environmental stewardship. Similarly, effective planning, communication, and collaboration strategies help mitigate untoward stress, such as that associated with unexpected change, software and equipment failure, and system and communications network downtime.

Integrated Functional Area Example: Telehealth and Informatics

Informatics solutions provide foundational support for healthcare delivery. In some cases, however, informatics solutions are more closely integrated with the delivery of care. This is particularly true for health care provided via telehealth services, where clinical care and informatics intersect in the provision of healthcare management.

Telehealth services are growing rapidly, with an expanding integration of health information technology into a variety of products. These products include tools used to provide direct patient care, but arc certainly not limited to healthcare provider services. A variety of health applications (*apps*), remote monitoring, contact-free monitoring apps, wearable health technology devices, mHealth, and other health and fitness devices are available to the consumer and are heavily marketed by new and developing companies using health information technology.

Such new tools and ideas are intended to provide increased access to needed health services, improve quality of care, and reduce the cost of associated healthcare services, all while focusing on the goal of improving patient outcomes. The explosively expanding use of telehealth services and products creates a need to develop and amend certain laws, rules, and regulations, especially related to licensure portability, to allow the full use of telehealth services by all practitioners for all people. Standards of care and best-practice recommendations for the use of telehealth services in a variety of specialties have been developed and revised (American Telemedicine Association [ATA], 2013), and should be incorporated in practices and in policies governing the use of telehealth services. The interface between nursing informatics and telehealth nursing is evolving with an increasing emphasis on the appropriate use and management of information and technology. Nursing informatics is used primarily to support clinical roles and is an essential component of the provision of telehealth services.

Nursing informatics supports multiple constituencies and stakeholders, such as healthcare consumers, interprofessional healthcare team members, IT professionals, and healthcare agencies and organizations. Informatics nurses are particularly well suited to work in such interprofessional environments, because of their preparation in the foundation of professional nursing focused on holistic patient, family, community, and population care and significant experience in planning, implementing, and coordinating activities involving multiple constituencies. With the continued developments in information science and nursing science, NI functions will continue to expand and evolve into functional areas not yet envisioned or recognized.

Evolution of Informatics Competencies

Because of the increased visibility of information and technology in healthcare settings and complementary educational programs, many stakeholders are faced with a need to define informatics competencies for every registered nurse, advanced practice registered nurse, and those who specialize in nursing Informatics practice. Managers, human resource managers, and educational planners are just three examples of stakeholders who have an interest in having defined competencies for nursing informatics.

Informatics Competencies Requisite for All Registered Nurses

The increasing complexity of healthcare services and practice, combined with the evolving mandate for ubiquitous electronic health information systems, has raised the bar for the nursing professional. Select informatics competencies are now required in all prelicensure, undergraduate, graduate, and doctoral nursing curricula. The National League for Nursing (NLN, 2008) advises nursing faculty to participate in programs to advance informatics development and to incorporate principles of informatics into each level of nursing curriculum. The American Association of Colleges of Nurses (AACN) identifies information management and the application of technology in patient care as an essential element of baccalaureate (AACN, 2008), master's (AACN, 2011), and doctor of nursing practice level (AACN, 2006) education. The Quality and Safety Education for Nurses (QSEN Institute, 2012a, 2012b; AACN, 2013) initiative has identified the nursing informatics competencies vital for the provision of safe, quality care to the public.

According to the Technology Informatics Guiding Education Reform (TIGER) initiative, all practicing nurses should be equipped with the skills necessary to practice in the technology-driven world of health care (Hebda & Calderone, 2010). A reference list of specific competencies needed by all practicing nurses was developed in 2009 by the Technology Informatics Guiding Education Reform group (TIGER, 2009). The TIGER initiative is "focused on using informatics tools, principles, theories and practices to enable nurses to make healthcare safer, more effective, efficient, patient-centered, timely and equitable" (TIGER, 2009, p. 2).

The TIGER Nursing Informatics Competencies Model is based on international standards such as the European Computer Driving License, the American Library Association Information Literacy Competency Standards; the Electronic Health Record Functional Model: Clinical Care Components, and the International Computer Driving License: Health (TIGER, 2009, p. 6). The TIGER model consists of three parts:

1. basic computer competencies

2. information literacy

3. information management (including use of an electronic health record)

Unlike some other lists of competencies, there are measurable competencies, such as:

- Know what computer memory is: RAM (random-access memory) and ROM (read-only memory), and distinguish between them or

- Use the components of a citation (e.g., currency, reputation of author or source, format, or elements of a URL) to choose those most suitable for the information need.

The complete *Informatics Competencies for Every Practicing Nurse: Recommendations from the TIGER Collaborative* report can be downloaded from http://www.thetigerinitiative.org/docs/TigerReport_ InformaticsCompetencies_000.pdf. Additional learning resources include the TIGER Virtual Learning Environment (available at http://www .thetigerinitiative.org/virtuallearning.aspx) and the government-funded Workforce Development Program (available at http://www.healthit.gov/policy -researchers-implementers/workforce-development-program; see also HealthIT Help Center Workforce Programs, n.d.).

Accredited graduate-level educational programs for the NI specialty nursing practice were first offered in 1989. Now graduate, doctoral, and postdoctoral degrees are more widely available via online and in-person learning programs. Lifelong learning can easily be accommodated by free nondegree online courses that offer open, unlimited, global enrollment massive open online courses (MOOCs) and other distance education and online programs. The current trend of requiring a graduate-level informatics degree is expected to continue and become the professional specialty practice standard.

Research About Nursing Informatics Competencies

In their seminal work on informatics competencies for nurses, Staggers, Gassert, and Curran (2001, 2002) studied the relationships between nursing roles and informatics competencies for nurses at four levels of practice: beginning, experienced, INS, and informatics innovator. This framework aligned with educational requirements for all nursing specialties at the beginning and experienced levels, and then identified specific competencies for the specialty roles of INS and the informatics innovator. The work of these authors not only promoted the integration of informatics competencies into educational curricula, but also influenced policy documents.

Since the 2008 publication of *Nursing Informatics: Scope and Standards of Practice*, research has progressed from determination to validation and implementation of nursing informatics competencies. Choi (2012) examined the informatics competencies of students in three undergraduate tracks: Traditional Pre-Licensure, Registered Nurse (RN) to Bachelor of Science in Nursing (BSN), and Accelerated BSN. Hsu et al. (2012) looked at the informatics competencies for mid-tier public health practitioners in the public health sector. Remus and Kennedy (2012) focused on the need for nursing informatics competencies in Canadian nurse leaders.

Other researchers continue to advance the work of Staggers, Gassert, and Curran. McGonigle, Hunter, Hebda, and Hill developed "a reliable and valid instrument for self-assessment of perceived level 3 informatics specialist and level 4 informatics innovator competencies in selected informatics activities" (2013, para. 4). Choi and Bakken (2013) reported on the validation of the self-assessment scale among undergraduate and graduate nursing students. Chang, Poynton, Gassert, and Staggers (2011) provided insight into the international use of Staggers, Gassert, and Curran's 2002 work. The ongoing work has been foundational in the development of this version of the nursing informatics scope and standards of practice.

Professional Organization Discussions on Informatics Competencies

Multiple organizations have provided input to the discussion on informatics competencies. This section provides an overview of several of these discussions.

HEALTHCARE LEADERSHIP ALLIANCE

The Healthcare Leadership Alliance (HLA) announced the creation of the HLA Competency Directory in the fall of 2005. This directory (HLA, 2005) identifies 300 competencies across multiple healthcare management roles, categorized into 5 domains:

- Leadership

- Communications and relationship management

- Professionalism

- Business knowledge and skills

- Knowledge of the healthcare environment

According to the web site (HLA, 2013, para. 4), the "directory provides a comprehensive listing of the competencies managers and leaders need to meet the challenges of managing the nation's healthcare organizations," including healthcare information management. These competencies may assist in the development and evaluation of informatics role definitions, including management roles.

AMERICAN ORGANIZATION OF NURSE EXECUTIVES

The American Organization of Nurse Executives, building on the mandate for informatics competencies for nurse leaders (AONE, 2005), demonstrated its support for informatics nurse leaders in the 2012 position paper "Nursing Informatics Executive Leader," which stated: "The NI Executive leader represents the bridge between clinical practice and informatics that transforms patient care delivery for the entire organization" (AONE, 2012, pg. 1).

QUALITY AND SAFETY EDUCATION FOR NURSES

The Quality and Safety Education for Nurses (QSEN) initiative project began in 2005 with the stated goal to "address the challenge of preparing future nurses with the knowledge, skills, and attitudes (KSAs) necessary to continuously improve the quality and safety of the healthcare systems in which they work" (QSEN Institute, 2012a, para. 1). QSEN has added informatics competences for prelicensure nursing education, based on work by Cronenwett et al. (2007), and for graduate nursing programs (QSEN Institute, 2012b).

NATIONAL LEAGUE FOR NURSING

In 2008, the National League for Nursing (NLN) released its position statement on preparing the next generation of nurses to be capable of functioning in a "technology rich environment" (NLN, 2008). To assist in that effort, NLN created tool kits for helping educators to assess their own competencies and provide teaching/learning strategies to assist with implementing informatics competencies into nursing education programs.

- NLN Informatics Education Toolkit (http://www.nln.org/facultyprograms/facultyresources/index.htm)

- NLN Competencies for Nursing Education (http://www.nln.org/facultyprograms/facultyresources/informatics.htm)

TIGER INITIATIVE FOUNDATION

The work of the original TIGER Initiative has been formalized with the establishment of a foundation that advances the integration of health informatics to transform practice, education, and consumer engagement, including the virtual learning environment (VLE). Ongoing results of the TIGER work can be found at http://www.thetigerinitiative.org/.

Informatics Competencies: Spanning Careers and Roles

Very few of today's nurses have worked in only one role or even one specialty of nursing throughout their careers, and this will likely hold true for coming generations of nurses. The need for informatics competencies exists in all nursing roles and specialties. This section examines the informatics competencies required for all practicing nurses, regardless of specialty.

The National Council of State Boards of Nursing (NCSBN) has developed and is studying a *Transition to Practice* (TTP) (Spector, 2013) nursing preceptor model that includes "five transition modules" consisting of "communication and teamwork, patient-centered care, evidence-based practice, quality improvement and informatics" (2013, para. 5). This model incorporates many key aspects from the Institute of Medicine's report on *The Future of Nursing: Leading Change, Advancing Health* (2010) related to competencies for all nurses, and "is an inclusive model, which would take place in all health care settings that hire newly graduated nurses and for all educational levels of nurses, including practical nurse, associate degree, diploma, baccalaureate and other entry-level graduates" (2013, para. 2). Because informatics and technology are now integral tools used in all aspects of nursing practice, from entry-level to advanced practice, it is strongly recommended that the state boards of nursing require that basic informatics competencies be incorporated into all nursing program curricula, ranging from licensed practical nurse (LPN) to doctoral levels.

As noted previously, the American Association of Colleges of Nursing (2008) provided guidance on the educational requirements for the baccalaureate education for professional nursing practice. "Essential IV: Information Management and Application of Patient Care Technology" identified informatics competencies that all BSN graduates should possess (pp. 1819). For nurses prepared at the graduate level, the AACN provided foundational informatics competencies in *The Essentials of Master's Education in Nursing*, "Essential V: Informatics and Healthcare Technologies" (2011, p. 19).

Nurses who hold a master's degree in something other than nursing can gain a postmaster's certificate in nursing informatics. Many of the numerous programs available have similar competencies, but in general the curricula focus on gaining specific knowledge and skills in nursing and healthcare informatics, thereby supporting evidence-based practice and the improvement of healthcare outcomes.

AACN's *Essentials of Doctoral Education for Advanced Nursing Practice* (2008) lists informatics-based competencies in "Essentials III: Clinical Scholarship and Analytical Methods for Evidence-Based Practice." Although only the Doctor of Nursing Practice (DNP) is specifically addressed by the AACN, this does not imply that informatics education is not important in PhD programs. In many PhD programs, computer science and biomedical informatics are required courses. However, because the DNP is considered a "practice doctorate" and the PhD a "nursing research doctorate," the emphasis on informatics and clinical *practice* impact is reduced, though these areas are not considered unimportant (AACN, 2011; see also Duke University, 2012). Thus, it is strongly recommended that PhD curriculum writers incorporate courses that examine the tenets of nursing informatics and focus on the methods of data entry, data storage, data retrieval, and data analysis from EHRs, report writing programs, and database management systems.

Informatics Competencies for Informatics Nurses and Informatics Nurse Specialists

In addition to the competencies that every registered nurse needs, additional competencies for the IN and INS are found in the "Standards of Nursing Informatics Practice" section of this professional resource. As part of its preparation for the new nursing informatics certification exam test form, the American Nurses Credentialing Center (ANCC) completed its *Role Delineation Study: Nursing Informatics—National Survey Results* (ANCC, 2013), which reported the collected information on the work activities that informatics nurses perform in practice. The final report listed 8 domains and 71 separate tasks, as well as calling out the 20 task statements with the highest and lowest values of initial risk.

The McGonigle, Hunter, Hebda, and Hill (2013) online assessment of nursing informatics competencies can assist faculty and management to develop curricula or continuing education that best meets the needs of their students or employees. While there are obvious concrete informatics competencies that every nurse must have, there are many other, more progressive, processes that will likely never be part of an educational curriculum or added to a formal list of competencies. An example is the ever-changing landscape of meaningful use criteria. Another example is the numerous ways in which technologies are enhancing practitioners' ability to monitor patients and coordinate care remotely via telehealth methodologies. All of these areas require informatics nurses and informatics nurse specialists to be involved in defining benefit versus impact, although it may be difficult to predict how the evolving technologies will be used in the future.

In addition to numerous researchers, academics, and employers, many professional organizations are actively working toward validating, creating resources, and providing education in nursing informatics. These include the:

- American Nurses Association (ANA)

- American Medical Informatics Association (AMIA)

- American Nursing Informatics Association (ANIA)

- Health Information and Management Systems Society (HIMSS) Nursing Informatics Working Group

Informatics Competencies for Nurse Educators

Today's nursing educators are challenged to include information on informatics in a basic nursing education curriculum that is already full. A second challenge is that many nurse educators themselves lack informatics competencies (AACN, 2013; Flood, Gasiewicz, & Delpier, 2010).

The Gordon and Betty Moore Foundation funded a pilot conference to teach faculty how to teach informatics. The "QSEN Nursing Informatics Deep Dive Workshop" was co-sponsored by the American Association of Colleges of Nursing and the Schools of Nursing at the Universities of Minnesota and Maryland. The presentations and resources are available to anyone, without charge, on the AACN website (http://www.aacn.nche.edu/qsen-informatics/2012-workshop).

Additional challenges include (1) continuing to enhance and disseminate resources and teaching strategies for all faculties across the country; (2) the lack of requirements for PhD programs in nursing to include informatics (researchers are going to need advanced informatics skills); and (3) the need for methods required for "big data" research to be integrated into curricula for future faculty and nurse researchers (Bickford, 2013, personal communication).

Office of the National Coordinator for Health Information Technology

In recognition of the need for health information technology specialists to assist providers in selecting, implementing, maintaining, and utilizing electronic medical record systems to "improve health care quality, safety, and cost-effectiveness" (HealthIT Help Center Workforce Programs, n.d., para. 1), and the need for those professionals to have specific competencies, the Office of the National Coordinator for Health Information Technology (ONC) sponsored four programs using American Recovery and Reinvestment Act funds. These four programs were:

- Curriculum Development Centers

- Community College Consortia to Educate Health Information Technology Professionals (Community College Consortia, n.d.)

- Program of Assistance for University-Based Training

- Competency Examination Program (HealthIT.gov, 2014)

The purpose of the Curriculum Development Centers Program was to fund and make resources available for curriculum building in higher education institutions. Under this program, the Oregon Health and Science Center was appointed to be the National Training and Dissemination Center (NTDC). Its task was to create a standard curriculum with competencies for all educators to use and students to understand and achieve (Curriculum Development Centers, n.d.).

Subsequently, the materials and curriculum created by the NTDC have been used by a community college consortium. This consortium consists of 82 member colleges in 5 regions across the United States. The program is focused on health care and IT professionals who want to become knowledgeable about and obtain jobs in the health IT sector. The following are key components of the curriculum:

- Practice workflow and information management redesign specialists

- Clinician/practitioner consultants

- Implementation support specialists

- Implementation managers

- Technical/software support

- Trainers

The materials were only available for download by consortia colleges through the end of 2012. Even though initial funding for the program has expired, most have commited to continuing their programs. As of February 2013, 17,523 health IT professionals had successfully completed the program, and 70% are working in the health IT field (HealthIT, 2013).

In addition to the community college consortium curriculum, funding was also allocated to develop university-based programs to increase the number of focused health IT professional roles. The six roles targeted by these programs are:

1. Clinician/public health leader

2. Health information management and exchange specialist

3. Health information privacy and security specialist

4. Research and development scientist

5. Programmer and software engineer

6. Health IT sub-specialist (Morton, 2011)

Lastly, the ONC funded the development and administration of a nationwide program of competency examinations. The purpose was to create "a mechanism to assess whether examinees have attained a certain set of health

IT competencies" (HealthIT.gov, 2014, para. 1). The project funding ended in April 2013, but the American Health Information Management Association (AHIMA) continues to administer the Certified in Healthcare Privacy and Security (CHPS®) and Certified Healthcare Technology Specialist (CHTS) examinations. To date, 9,527 health IT professionals have taken this examination (HealthIT.gov, 2014; see also CHPS, 2014; CHTS, 2013). The resources from these federally funded initiatives remain available in the public domain and have garnered signficant national and international interest and use.

Synthesis of Evolution of NI Competencies

After the initial work of Staggers et al. (2002), numerous authors and agencies published work on informatics competencies. The focus of the work on informatics competencies over the past five years has changed from determining informatics competencies to validation and implementation. The TIGER Initiative's work has provided specific and measureable criteria.

Multiple professional organizations are supporting the call for nursing and healthcare informatics competencies as a part of professional practice. Figure 6 depicts the need for informatics education in all levels of nursing, from both

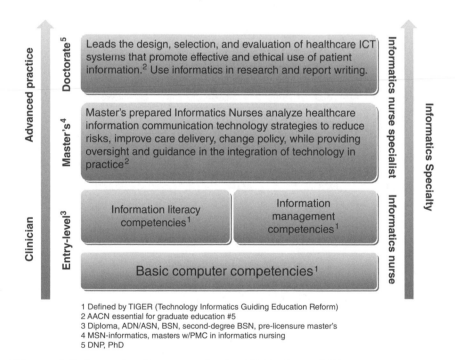

1 Defined by TIGER (Technology Informatics Guiding Education Reform)
2 AACN essential for graduate education #5
3 Diploma, ADN/ASN, BSN, second-degree BSN, pre-licensure master's
4 MSN-informatics, masters w/PMC in informatics nursing
5 DNP, PhD

Figure 6. Informatics Competencies for All Registered Nurses

the clinical and educational points of view, as well as for those nurses who specialize in informatics. Informatics education must be foundational for all entry-level nurses. Over time, as their education, knowledge, and skills increase, nurses grow in their understanding of how to use technology to enable them to provide better patient care. Finally, as newer and better ways of using technology (innovation) emerge, nurses who specialize in informatics nursing will have a leading role.

In the future, the rapid pace of technological change and generation of information and knowledge will present challenges for the maintenance of current and accurate competencies for nursing informatics. Nurses must understand the need for achieving basic competence in nursing informatics; professional organizations must continue to embrace informatics as a foundation for professional practice; and faculty must make NI an integral part of curricula at all levels of nursing education, as well as stimulate continued research. It is the responsibility of informatics nurses to be the resource for these initiatives.

Preparation for Nursing Informatics Specialty Practice

The following exemplifies one pathway for the novice nurse to move from an entry-level informatics nurse job to a position deemed to be a true informatics nurse leader, regardless of formal title. At any time in their careers, nurses interested in health information technology could complete one or all of the ONC community college consortia programs and pass the associated certification exam to become a health information technology specialist, thus becoming better able to function in and attain positions in academic, clinical practice, administrative, and technology areas.

Because nursing informatics requires a significant understanding of numerous clinical workflows, it is advisable for an aspiring informatics nurse to spend at least five years at the bedside or in other clinical practice experiences in numerous departments and roles. As aspiring informatics nurses continue to educate themselves through formal programs or through informatics-focused areas of practice, they will become more comfortable in taking on greater levels of responsibility and accountability reflective of nursing informatics practice. Becoming a subject matter expert for a specialty role, whether academic, clinical, or administrative, will further enhance the nurse's understanding of the nuances involved in developing, maintaining, and optimizing technology that impacts nursing in all realms.

Since 2004, the Health Information and Management Systems Society (HIMSS) has surveyed the nursing informatics community to gain an understanding of the roles and responsibilities of the informatics nurse professional. The most recent *Nursing Informatics Workforce Survey* (HIMSS, 2014), supported by the HIMSS Nursing Informatics Community, representing 6,000 nurses, builds on previous HIMSS research from 2004, 2007, and 2011. This survey captures current professional status and practice trends while identifying changes that have occurred over the past nine years in the nursing informatics workforce. The 1,047 respondents reported that 60% had completed graduate or higher degree educational preparation, 58% worked at a hospital, and 13% worked at the corporate offices of a healthcare system; the average salary was $100,717. (Further details are available at http://www.himss.org/ni-workforce-survey.)

Certification of Informatics Nurses

Professional certification as an informatics nurse became a reality in late 1995 when the American Nurses Credentialing Center offered the generalist-level nursing informatics certification exam as its first computer-based examination. As of December 31, 2013, the ANCC reported that 1,326 nurses have active credentials of board certification in nursing informatics. Applicants currently must have at least a BSN or baccalaureate degree in another related area, have completed the specified continuing education credits, and have worked in informatics practice for the designated number of hours. (More details are available at www.nursecredentialing.org.) Informatics nurses and informatics nurse specialists may elect to pursue other pertinent certifications in areas such as project management, security and privacy, health information systems management, network management, and knowledge management. Employers are beginning to move from a preference to a requirement for certification for hiring, advancement, and promotion decisions.

An Advancing Professional Nursing Specialty

The blending of clinical background, on-the-job training, refined and focused informatics competencies, informatics certification, and the increase in formalized informatics education are proof of an advancing professional nursing specialty that is ideally suited to lead in an informatics-based U.S. healthcare system. Employers are beginning to recognize the value and contribution of informatics nurses and are even requiring completion of graduate or higher level educational preparation for hiring. Similarly, the informatics nurse specialist title is becoming more familiar. As the importance of nursing informatics continues to be recognized, the future should see a rise in executive-level or C-Suite nursing informatics positions, such as "Chief Nursing Informatics Officer," in clinical, business, vendor, and IT arenas. In addition, the need for nursing informatics professionals in governmental roles will be recognized at the local, state, regional, and national levels. Nurses with an interest in informatics have many avenues through which to pursue their specialty practice over the years.

Ethics in Nursing Informatics

Code of Ethics for Nurses (ANA, 2001) provides a framework for ethical practice in nursing informatics. While working in the informatics role, professional nurses may not provide direct patient care, but do provide support for patient care through work on the healthcare delivery system infrastructure through which care is delivered. All provisions of this Code apply to nursing informatics— some more directly than others, as illustrated in the following examples.

Provision 1: The nurse, in all professional relationships, practices with compassion and respect for the inherent dignity, worth and uniqueness of every individual, unrestricted by considerations of social or economic status, personal attributes, or the nature of health problems.

The informatics nurse and informatics nurse specialist function as integral parts of the healthcare team. The nature of this work involves interaction and collaboration with many different people with various areas of expertise, values, priorities, and views. The informatics nurse values each of these people as individuals, with worth and dignity, regardless of status or power in the organization, and in spite of some persons' lack of informatics or nursing knowledge. The team collaboration that is essential to successful information systems in health care is created, enhanced, and preserved through the informatics nurse's compassion and respect for each person on the team.

Provision 2: The nurse's primary commitment is to the patient, whether an individual, family, group or community.

The informatics nurse always works to achieve results that will directly or indirectly benefit patient care, safety, and well-being. This involves careful consideration of the probable outcomes of decisions about data collection and protection of the privacy, security, and confidentiality of patient information. The informatics nurse avoids participating in the development or implementation of systems that may be desired by an interested party, but that would have the effect of causing harm to the patient. For example, countering such adverse effects may require the development of an effective system alert that directs a clinician to offer less costly and comparable alternatives for medications or treatments.

Provision 3: The nurse promotes, advocates for and strives to protect the health, safety and rights of the patient.

As the patient advocate, the informatics nurse collaborates in the development, implementation, support, and maintenance of systems with data collection, storage, retrieval, processing, and analytic features that support: (a) patient safety, autonomy, and rights; (b) quality improvement efforts; (c) provision of safe care; (d) appropriate information communication; (e) restriction of access to patient data by those not authorized to have it; and (f) use of data and information to benefit healthcare outcomes and healthcare services delivery. The informatics nurse is involved in addressing usability factors that support the rights of the patient.

Provision 4: The nurse is responsible and accountable for individual nursing practice and determines the appropriate delegation of tasks consistent with the nurse's obligation to provide optimum patient care.

The informatics nurse uses best practices in informatics to collaborate in the development, implementation, support, and maintenance of systems that support nursing practice. The informatics nurse supports direct care providers in their efforts to learn about, understand, and use information technology in a way that supports patient care and promotes the patient's welfare.

Provision 5: The nurse owes the same duties to self as to others, including the responsibility to preserve integrity and safety, to maintain competence, and to continue personal and professional growth.

The informatics nurse is responsible for maintaining currency in informatics theory and practice through lifelong learning. This can be challenging in a field with rapidly changing technologies and capabilities and a fiscally constrained environment that requires self-funding of relevant continuing education programs and activities. For a more detailed discussion of lifelong learning and maintenance of competence, see Professional Performance Standard 8, Education.

Provision 6: The nurse participates in establishing, maintaining, and improving healthcare environments and conditions of employment conducive to the provision of quality healthcare and consistent with the values of the profession through individual and collective action.

The informatics nurse collaborates in the development, implementation, support, and maintenance of information systems that support and improve the delivery of care, appropriate communication of health-related information, data storage, protection of confidential information, and management of the enterprise. Such behavior provides a model for successful interprofessional teams.

Provision 7: The nurse participates in the advancement of the profession through contributions to practice, education, administration, and knowledge development.

Informatics nurses seek to advance the quality of nursing informatics practice. As a specialty, nursing informatics offers both master's and doctoral degrees in which students can gain the advanced nursing education necessary to add to the body of informatics knowledge, and the credentials to teach informatics to the next generations of nurses. Informatics nurse specialists are prepared to improve administration, education, and research in nursing informatics, and to enhance dissemination of that knowledge.

Provision 8: The nurse collaborates with other health professionals and the public in promoting community, national, and international efforts to meet health needs.

The informatics nurse collaborates in efforts to develop systems that allow system interoperability and data and information transfer and aggregation. These efforts allow health data to be used to improve knowledge about individual, community, national, and international health and health practices and outcomes.

Provision 9: The profession of nursing, as represented by associations and their members, is responsible for articulating nursing values, for maintaining the integrity of the profession and its practice, and for shaping social policy.

The informatics nurse participates in the informatics work of professional nursing associations, in national and international health informatics organizations, and in vendor organizations, to articulate nursing values, to ensure that patient-centricity is always maintained, and to shape social and health policy for the benefit of all persons.

The Future of Nursing Informatics

Five trends will continue to influence the future of nursing informatics: (1) changing practice roles in nursing, (2) increasing informatics competence requirements for all nurses, (3) rapidly evolving technology, (4) regulatory changes and quality standards that include healthcare consumers as partners in healthcare models, and (5) care delivery models and innovation.

Trends in Practice Roles and Competencies for Nurses and Informatics

The principles of evidence-based practice and application of technologies are now being integrated into the workplace in all settings. This results in the need for every nurse to have some level of informatics competence, with the number and complexity of informatics competencies evolving to meet their changing practice roles. As discussed earlier, some of the basic informatics competencies once ascribed to informatics specialists have become mandatory for nurses in clinical, education, and administration practices. Similarly, the level of competencies required for INs and INSs has increased to meet the skill-set requirements necessary to participate on the development and implementation teams.

In the past several years, nursing specialties have incorporated informatics into their practice. For example, nurses who rely on information and technology for telehealth, quality improvement, or product development might be considered informatics nurses. Other nurses who design, implement, and evaluate informatics solutions as active members of the interprofessional teams are acting in very common nursing informatics roles. The scope of nursing informatics practice will continue to expand as further technologic innovations are developed for healthcare delivery solutions. Nursing informatics has become a world community.

The role boundaries between other health informatics roles and NI are less conspicuous than in the past. One of the centerpieces of nursing informatics practice is its interprofessional nature, with informatics nurse specialists often leading projects to craft usable informatics solutions for use by many stakeholders. Although INSs focus on technology and nursing practice, they work in teams with informatics specialists from other healthcare professions such as medicine, pharmacy, and respiratory therapy. These interprofessional teams are using a shared set of functions, skills, and their knowledge of their respective professions to craft solutions that meet the needs of all. This trend will likely continue as professional informatics organizations define a shared set of core knowledge and skills required by all informatics specialties.

Probably the clearest trend is ongoing change in the functional areas for informatics nurses and informatics nurse specialists, moving from a generic set of skills toward a shared set of competencies based on functional areas required to enact a particular position (e.g., clinical analyst, informatics executive, futurist, knowledge discovery and data mining [KDD] researcher, database developer).

Trends in Technology

Information technology has become commonplace in everyone's personal lives, as well as in delivery of healthcare services. For the first time in history, a generation exists that has never known a world without the Internet, cell phones, online social networks, blogs, and other electronic media. People who were raised using this technology (*digital natives*) are now entering the healthcare field as knowledge workers, as well as consumers of healthcare services. Implications for nursing informatics include:

- New models of work and education for technologically sophisticated users who are less resistant to technology and in fact demand it.

- Adapting to users with less skill in face-to-face communications.

- Consumers with even greater expectations of accelerated information and technology implementation.

Several advances in technology will likely have an impact on nursing informatics in the future. A number of these are outlined in the following subsections.

NANOTECHNOLOGY

Nanotechnology is microscopic technology on the order of one-billionth of a meter. The application of this technology for healthcare delivery uses (nano-medicine) will have an impact on the diagnosis and treatment of many diseases and conditions (Jain, 2008; Maojo et al., 2011). For example, these minute biomedical devices (smaller than molecules) are being developed to provide a way to deliver therapies (medication and radiation) that will target cancer cells or that can perform surgery (nanorobots) on specific cells. The implementation of this technology for patient care applications requires education in its safe use as well as ethical practices (McGonigle & Mastrian, 2015, p. 485; see also http://www.nano.gov/ and http://www.ihe.ca/publications/library/2012-publications/exploratory-brief-on-nanomedicine-or-the-appliation-of-nanotechnology-in-human-health-care/).

TOOLS FOR MANAGING POPULATION HEALTH CONCERNS

As healthcare delivery moves into the global community setting, there will be a growing need for informatics support for disease state management and population health activities (e.g., public health, school health, and occupational health). Informatics provides tools that allow data collection, analysis, and reporting of population health specialty data by the use of standardized variables in interoperable electronic documentation systems (see http://www.ncqa.org/HEDISQualityMeasurement.aspx and http://www.dartmouthatlas.org/). Population health specialty data then become a useful tool to support research, inform policy, and identify best practices to enhance treatment of national population health concerns.

Syndromic surveillance of communicable disease using school absenteeism records (Baer, Rodriguez, & Duchin, 2011), and management of immunization data (Hinman & Ross, 2010), each provide insight into the potential of population-level data. School health and public health nurses are leading movements to standardize variables and data collection processes that will enhance this ability. This potential for research and analysis is exemplified in the data collected by school nurses on more than 95% of the school-aged population. Other examples of this potential will be driven by business globalization and the threat of bioterrorism. The desire for improved disease management across traditional boundaries will lead to a demand for new population health tools and solutions.

The need for population management tools and early disease detection has led to partnerships with population health professionals and the emergence of public health informatics (Public Health Informatics Institute [PHII], 2009). MappyHealth and other geographic information system (GIS) applications are being implemented as strategies to support syndromic surveillance, emergency preparedness, and disaster recovery efforts. Health information exchanges and disease and immunization registries help identify and address public health concerns.

DEVICES AND HARDWARE

The miniaturization of devices has changed where and how IT solutions can be deployed. No perfect hardware solution exists. However, technological innovations are making headway in meeting changing healthcare delivery models, particularly the caregiver needs for the older adult population. An increasing focus on ergonomics, human–computer interaction, and user experience is leading to new solutions to support diverse workflow requirements.

New integrated technologies, such as smartphones, tablets, and multifunctional devices, have increased common access to health information. These solutions are becoming ubiquitous in daily life. They have changed clinicians' and patients' expectations and their interactions with technology. In particular, providers are being challenged to know as much about new disease treatments and research findings as patients.

Some of the pending technologies that will affect INs, INSs, clinicians, patients, and healthcare consumers include:

New methods for medication administration

- Sensing a patient's internal drug levels with miniature medical diagnostic tools circulating in the patient's bloodstream.

- Chemotherapy delivered directly to a tumor site, reducing systemic side effects.

New monitoring devices and miniaturization for the home that move content to hardware and devices

- A talking pill bottle that lets patients push a button to hear prescription information.

- Bathroom counters that announce whether it is safe to mix two medications.

- A shower with built-in scales to calculate body mass index (Hong Kong Polytechnic University).

■ Measuring devices in the bathroom to track urination frequency and output and upload these data to a system or care manager.

■ Noninvasive blood glucose monitors to eliminate fingersticks; sensors to compute blood sugar levels using a multi-wavelength reflective dispersion photometer (Hong Kong Polytechnic University).

Body area network (wearable computing)

■ Wearable computing, or body-borne computing, will continue to evolve in the next several years and have an impact similar to that of mobile computing on our daily lives. Innovations in development involve eyeglasses or clothing that interact with the user based on the context of the situation. With heads-up displays, sensors embedded in fabrics, unobtrusive input devices, personal wireless local area networks, and a host of other context-sensing and communication tools, wearable computers can act as intelligent assistants or data collection and analysis devices.

Many of these devices are available now. Smart fabrics with embedded sensors have been on the commercial market since 2000 and are being used in shirts, gloves, and other clothing. These wearable computer and remote monitoring systems are intertwined with the user's activity so that the technology becomes transparent. Sensors and devices can gather data during the patient's daily routine, providing healthcare providers or researchers with periodic or continuous data on the subject's health at work, school, exercise, and sleep, rather than the current snapshot captured during a typical hospital or clinic visit. A few applications for wearable computing include:

■ Monitoring rescue workers' vital signs, heat stress, and dehydration

■ Activity level of poststroke patients

■ Assessment of stress in individuals

■ Arrhythmia detection and control of selected cardiac conditions

■ Daily activity monitors

■ Proximity badges and RFID (radio-frequency identification) to track providers for workflow or allow logon to systems.

■ Glasses with a heads-up display that can superimpose images (e.g., chest x-ray) in a display over a patient, without losing focus on the patient (MIT Media Lab, 2012).

■ Bar-code scanners that fit on a finger, or wrist-activated input devices.

Developments for input methods also apply to the healthcare market. For example, an "interface-free," touch-driven computer screen, manipulated intuitively with the fingertips, responds to varying levels of pressure. Another example is virtual keyboards using Bluetooth technology, in which a keyboard can be displayed and used on any surface (*ThinkGeek*, 2014).

ROBOTICS

The use of robotics in patient care has also revolutionized health care. Robots continue to be used to deliver supplies to patient care areas, enable remote surgeries and virtual-reality surgical procedure training, and are being used as translators for patients. Hand-assist devices help patients regain strength after a stroke, and robotic technology is being used for immediate patient assessments (Leventhal, 2010).

Robots are providing a remote presence by allowing clinicians to virtually examine patients by manipulating remote cameras. Robotics are also being used in direct patient care: for instance, to help lift morbidly obese patients, to assist patients who have had traumatic injuries, and in other innovative applications (Robotics Technology-Healthcare Robotics, n.d.). A notable use is the research underway for using robotics to assist paralyzed patients to walk (Houlihan, n.d.).

FOCUS OF EMERGING TECHNOLOGIES

Clinicians are using new and evolving technologies to deliver care that results in decreased barriers, increased access, improved outcomes, and increased patient engagement in their own health. Telehealth tools and emerging technologies are positioned to change the face and practice of health care. Nurses using informatics, telehealth tools, and new, transformative technologies will be well positioned to interact with and care for their patients virtually. There will be a decreasing number of brick-and-mortar practices and an increasing number of clinicians and specialists available—for a fraction of traditional costs—at the click of a button.

Gaming technology has entered the healthcare arena as well. Health and fitness apps and devices are being marketed to consumers as products that can be used to monitor actions and activities that affect health status. The use of creative health-related technology with social media integration may increase patient engagement and improve wellness.

Virtual worlds are being created (e.g., Second Life©) that allow consumers to interact with providers to seek care at a distance. The Department of Defense is using avatars to help veterans with posttraumatic stress disorder (PTSD) (Hemmerly-Brown, 2011). Practices are being developed completely online in the virtual world that allow patients to create an avatar and seek health care while concealing their physical identity. Nursing informatics involvement is needed to bridge solutions that support virtual health worlds as well as complement face-to-face care with virtual care.

Healthcare education and research can be conducted within a virtual world (Wisconsin Institute for Discovery, n.d.). Software programs have been developed to assist nursing and medical students to learn physical assessment via simulated practice with a digital patient, document in an electronic medical records system, and explore medical concepts in three dimensions in a virtual world (Shadow Health, 2014).

Remote monitoring, mHealth devices and hardware, other devices creating "smart" homes, and other digital solutions will continue to be developed and improved. Healthcare professionals who use these emerging technologies will need to be equipped with knowledge of rules, regulations, and responsibilities surrounding the use of these technologies. Patients and clinicians alike will need education on how to use, share, and benefit from the "big data" that are produced and gathered by these devices.

Health-related education will move online with more frequency as providers learn to interact with their patients virtually. Holograms are being utilized to provide health education and serve as virtual coaches (Bassendowski, 2013). Software has been developed that allows providers to choose a diagnosis and allows the computer to provide structured educational programs for the patient. Technology is also moving more toward a semantic web, in which technological programs will actually interact with patients, learn their needs, and adjust education based upon the patients' responses.

New technology is being used to provide telecommunication connectivity where broadband is not available. This allows specialists and other healthcare providers to interact with those in need in rural communities, decreases barriers related to transportation, and facilitates implementation of best practices for vulnerable populations where access to health care was previously limited or unavailable.

Goals related to care will remain the same in regard to decreasing hospital admissions, improving outcomes, and keeping patients healthy at home and in their local community. However, the methods for accomplishing these goals may change as an understanding of the use and benefits of telehealth and emerging technologies becomes more widespread.

KNOWLEDGE REPRESENTATION

Electronic data are now available for and about patients over their lifetime. Clinicians need tools to help locate and synthesize these data remotely and securely. Innovative technology is being used to allow the wireless display (via smartphones, tablets, laptops, etc.) of data to clinicians to optimize patient care and enhance patient and clinician efficiencies, while avoiding medical errors. NI practice now requires that more nurses be educated about knowledge representation, semantic representation, and other knowledge areas, including use of standardized language that supports nursing practice and decision-making. This also has implications for knowledge discovery in databases, data quality, and a continued emphasis on data standards and data quality.

Nurses constantly make complex and diverse decisions in their daily practice. Decision-making must consider relevant evidence-based and patient-specific information. As nurse decision-making becomes more complex, the need for computerized clinical decision support will increase. In the absence of explicit evidence-based guidelines for nursing decisions, novel technologies will be necessary to synthesize evidence from the literature or induce models from clinical data.

Knowledge discovery in databases could play an important role in the induction of clinical knowledge models. Informatics nurses must partner in the planning of and forward thinking about maintenance and evaluation of legacy data, mandates for interoperability, and data conversion and retention, as well as accessibility for future use.

EDUCATIONAL TECHNOLOGIES

Evolving teaching technologies are changing the education techniques used in the classroom, the lab, and the clinical setting. For example, patient care simulation activities allow students to run programmed care scenarios in a safe environment and provide innovative options for teaching and fostering critical thinking skills (Sternberger, 2012). Group learning tools, such as electronic reminders and group scoring used in interactive teaching, can change how students engage with class content, as well as how they learn to function as members of a team (Michaelsen, n.d.).

Distance education technologies, and web-based and cloud-based collaboration (such as web-based course management systems and the related student support services), are challenging basic education concepts such as what academic resources must be included in a library collection or how a university defines a credit hour of education. This automation is forcing institutions to review, and in many cases to revise, their educational policies and procedures. These technologies require a paradigm shift in knowledge delivery, which affects students, instructors, and course content, and create significant opportunities for innovative informatics nurses.

The traditional tuition models are no longer a barrier to the globalization of education. New educational models are being created, such as global universities that reach students beyond their walls by offering courses on location or by creating virtual educational experiences (e.g., partnering with other institutions to deliver classes to students across a region). Universities are also partnering with business entities and vendors to create other innovative models of education (Emory University, 2011).

Curriculum design will change. The traditional classroom is also changing to the concept of the *flipped classroom* model, which permits interactive collaboration in the classroom (Brame, 2013). Information is now generated and made available so quickly that baseline knowledge for students will evolve away from specific content to methods of finding accurate, current information and knowledge. Future students may not be evaluated on specific knowledge for one area or course, but instead be evaluated on their growth over time. The INS will be at the center of this union of informatics and new educational models because of the INS role's focus on managing information.

TOOLS FOR PATIENT ACCESS TO HEALTH INFORMATION

Much emphasis is being placed on assisting healthcare consumers to become partners with their providers, thereby increasing consumers' accountability for their own care. The healthcare consumers may be known as e-patients (e-Patients.net, 2013). This type of healthcare model will require clinical nurses and informatics nurses to devise personalized solutions and the best methods of care and patient education, as well as solutions to monitor and maintain patients' health. Patient engagement is expected to include easy access to personal health information via the view, download, and transmit (VDT) capabilities being mandated by the ONC for meaningful use compliance. Surrounding issues that must be addressed include: healthcare consumer-centered care/patient-centered care, patient accountability for care activities and data integrity, interoperable data transfer, education about data protection and security, and medical identity theft and encryption tools that monitor and protect.

EXPANDED USE OF IT IN NURSING

Technologic innovation has had an enormous impact on the scope of nursing practice in traditional work settings, in the home, and globally. Two implications are outlined here. One is a concern about students relying on available, structured information, computerized alerts, and reminders in EHRs and decision-support systems (DSSs). Some educators and administrators are concerned that students will rely only on this structured information rather than applying their critical thinking skills, and that those skills may thus diminish. INSs and educators are developing and testing new academic and practice models that address this issue. One solution involves the development of case studies that can be used in simulated settings and include the integrated use of EHRs with DSSs. System designers may need to modify systems to promote a different cognitive engagement by practitioners. Educators may teach a new level of human information processing to enhance thoughtful decision-making. The traditional model involves students memorizing structures for a physical examination and similar static information stored in an EHR. In the new model, information technology serves as an aid to, not a replacement for, human thinking and judgment, to promote collaborative patient management.

Reliability is the other implication of the increasing pervasiveness of IT. As applications are increasingly integrated into health care, the impact of downtime or system unavailability becomes more severe and quick recovery methods become imperative. Especially with order management in place, institutions must ensure continuous business operations with uninterrupted access to applications and data. Strategies and technologies to support continuous uptime are available, and the INS is typically involved in defining, designing, and installing them. Requirements for current and future systems will focus more on proactive risk mitigation rather than reactive recovery efforts; these may include:

- 24/7 operation and performance with redundancies throughout the system, failovers, and tested high reliability.

- Tools to assist in monitoring and managing the IT environment, monitor system use, and identify technology issues before system failure occurs.

- Scalable IT solutions as more clinical applications come online.

- Solutions that IT departments can manage without in-depth technology expertise.

- Implementation of health information exchanges (HIEs) to facilitate the sharing of patient information.

IMPLICATIONS FOR NURSING INFORMATICS

Informatics nurses will need a systematic method for becoming aware of emerging technologies and tools and then evaluating their usability for and projected impact(s) on health care and informatics. INs and INSs can be essential leaders and partners for the safe and intelligent incorporation of new technology and techniques into health informatics solutions and health care in general. Because the content or information on devices is still the most critical component, informatics nurses can serve as content designers. Areas such as genomics have significant ethical ramifications, and informatics nurses must ensure that attention is given to these issues. All of these areas have implications for curricular design and educational programming as well.

The expansion of technology amplifies the need for continuous availability of systems. Nevertheless, the "digital divide" remains, as significant numbers of people have little access to or experience with information technology. Informatics nurses can also take the lead in eliminating the digital divide between those with access to information and those without. In all situations, informatics nurses can advocate and apply methods so that users can learn and use new technologies effectively and safely.

Trends in Regulatory Changes and Quality Standards

Technologies cannot remain the primary focus when addressing the future of nursing informatics and health care. The design and evolution of healthcare systems, organizations, and enterprises, as well as the regulatory environment and actual models of care delivery, must be integral and primary considerations.

The 2009 American Recovery and Reinvestment Act (ARRA) and Health Information Technology for Economic and Clinical Health (HITECH) Act have driven information technology and EHR installations in the United States to a new national level, emphasizing the use of technology for patient safety and error reduction in healthcare delivery. Organizations such as the Agency for Healthcare Research and Quality (AHRQ) and the Institute for Healthcare Improvement (IHI), as well as nonhealth organizations like Leapfrog, provide incentives for health institutions to implement informatics solutions. The continuing requirement to meet meaningful use standards is supporting the increasing pace of adoption. Mandates now direct organizations to use value-based rather than return-on-investment models to justify health IT, and the pay-for-performance models are accelerating EHR installations. Online quality data and reported metrics are more visible to both consumers and hospital and organizational boards. Organizations will continue to increase the transparency of data and, more importantly, improve the care being delivered.

Regulatory requirements and standards will continue to shape the future. INSs are involved in defining these and future standards, and in designing, building, implementing, using, and certifying products that comply. A number of projects have been implemented; among them are the following:

- HL7 continues to define interoperability standards for systems.

- The IEEE P2407 working group has developed standards for personalized health informatics.

- The Healthcare Information Technology Standards Panel (HITSP) is harmonizing industry-wide health IT standards.

- The Nationwide Health Information Network (NwHIN) initiative is creating prototype architectures for widespread health information exchange.

- The Food and Drug Administration (FDA) initiatives related to (a) barcode label requirements for human drug products and biological products, (b) guidelines for the safe and effective use of radio frequency devices, and (c) nanotechnology development and potential expansion of products covered (e.g., advanced decision support tools and similar informatics applications).

- Office of the National Coordinator for Health Information Technology's *Connecting Health and Care for the Nation* concept paper (HealthIT. gov, n.d.).

Trends in Care Delivery Models and Innovation

Using technologies in new ways and inventing new technologies to enable better care delivery models to achieve quality outcomes and safety are part of the evolution to accountable care organizations (ACOs), a population focus rather than individual focus, and pay-for-performance rather than fee-for-service reimbursement. Care is no longer a local phenomenon. Patients in rural ICUs can be monitored remotely by intensivists and ICU nurses. Less experienced critical care nurses can be remotely mentored by experienced nurses. Pharmacists can provide remote pharmacologic assistance to rural areas. Radiologists can read images in real time from anywhere in the world. Physicians are assisted by robots as they examine patients in distant locations.

Care is no longer limited to traditional healthcare settings, even when it is delivered locally. Clinicians are now available in retail stores, work settings, and other nontraditional places. These new settings require new design, deployment, and support models that will challenge the informatics nurse specialist. Involvement in the development of a robust health information infrastructure includes, but is not limited to:

- Continued innovation in systems and expansion into less traditional settings, such as long-term care and rural communities.

- ACOs, medical home, home health expansion, and patient-aligned care teams (interprofessional team completing care coordination/management).

- Growth of personal health records. PHRs are more numerous and the use of the patient portal (PP) is being implemented along with electronic medical record (EMR) activations. Informatics nurses will increasingly advocate for and assist patients with developing these individually maintained records. These can include the patient's own electronic vaccination history, past medical history, medications, allergies, condition, status, and visit history in an easily accessible online format. Patients' online communication with healthcare providers through PPs will continue to increase as well.

- Clinical data repositories and regional health information organizations/exchanges. These structures will support accurate, timely, and secure transfer of patient data across care settings (ultimately across hospitals, clinics, pharmacies, laboratories, clinician office, long-term care facilities, and others).

Consumer Informatics

Healthcare consumers have become stronger partners with providers, embracing increased accountability for their own care and taking greater interest in data accuracy and access to their own electronic health information. As consumers become more technically adept, they will consider their electronic healthcare data as necessary and accessible as their online banking information or stock transactions. Likewise, consumers will begin monitoring and managing the health of younger *and* older family members for whom they are responsible.

In response to the increasing technology capabilities of healthcare consumers, the Centers for Medicare & Medicaid Services created Physician Compare (https://data.medicare.gov/data/physician-compare) and Hospital Compare (http://www.medicare.gov/hospitalcompare/) to help healthcare consumers select appropriate care delivery resources.

External Partnerships

Nontraditional organizations are now entering the healthcare arena, and their contributions and innovations should be welcomed. For example, companies with an online application for individual, secure financial records may expand their apps to include personal health records. Partnerships with the video-gaming industry yield ideas for optimal user interfaces and contribute to the development of healthcare and clinician educational media, products, and systems. Nurses need to be participants in this space, ideally as information and facility architects.

Implications for Nursing Informatics

New care delivery models will require development of informatics solutions for care in multiple, remote locations. Informatics nurses will have a key role in informatics solutions that emphasize quality care metrics developed as e-measures. New models to shorten the time from design to installation in the system life cycle are being used. An 18- to 24-month build-and-implementation cycle is not tenable in an era of rapidly changing technology, care delivery, and expanding information access.

With the increasing number of information technology installations and the need to respond to burgeoning regulatory requirements, informatics nurses are on center stage for all phases of the system life cycle. They are developing and implementing new informatics solutions, ensuring data quality for implemented solutions, and evaluating the impact of solutions. The new model of consumer informatics requires technical solutions and patient education jointly from clinical nurses and INSs. INSs will need to devise the best methods of care and also design solutions that enable patients to monitor and maintain their own health. INSs will play a key role in designing new tools for data capture and analyses to comply with regulatory guidelines.

NI Future and Trends: Summary

The practice of nursing, expanding competencies, technologic innovations, and new trends in healthcare delivery models and regulation will continue to influence the future of nursing informatics. Important concepts will be essential to these trends:

- Preparing for technology innovations, evidence-based practice competencies, and data quality evaluation.

- Introducing and delivering new educational models to teach both new and existing nursing professionals.

- Designing, developing, implementing, and evaluating solutions for innovative information technologies across all areas of nursing and health settings.

- Incorporating telehealth and newer technologies and methods to facilitate access and care provision, research, and administrative processes.

- Designing and facilitating changes in care models in response to evidence-based practice outcomes as they evolve away from episodic care toward more predictive and preventive models with collaborative interprofessional care teams.

- Focusing on usability, designing and evaluating how information is presented to promote ease of use and adoption (human-computer interaction).

- Participating in global public and private initiatives to evaluate disease patterns and trends.

In the future, care models and data will continue to be shared even more widely. New technologies will create wider access to information and the need for a new generation of data and information management skills, analytic tools, educational models, and cognitive skills. Traditional boundaries of institutions, care delivery, and education will continue to shift and evolve. New positions and functional areas are emerging. Increased collaboration among nursing informatics colleagues and a shared scope and standards of practice will continue to be a characteristic of the future.

Standards of Nursing Informatics Practice

Significance of the Standards

The *Standards of Professional Nursing Practice*, on which the Standards of Nursing Informatics Practice are based, are authoritative statements of the duties that all registered nurses, regardless of role, population, or specialty, are expected to perform competently. The standards published herein may be utilized as evidence of the standard of care, with the understanding that application of the standards is context dependent. The standards are subject to change with the dynamics of the nursing profession, as new patterns of professional practice are developed and accepted by the nursing profession and the public. In addition, specific conditions and clinical circumstances may affect the application of the standards at a given time (e.g., during a natural disaster). The standards are subject to formal, periodic review and revision.

The competencies that accompany each standard may be evidence of compliance with the corresponding standard. The list of competencies is not exhaustive. Whether a particular standard or competency applies depends on the circumstances.

Standards of Practice for Nursing Informatics

Standard 1. Assessment

The informatics nurse collects comprehensive data, information, and emerging evidence pertinent to the situation.

COMPETENCIES

The informatics nurse:

- Uses evidence-based assessment techniques, instruments, tools, and effective communication strategies in collecting pertinent data to define the issue or problem.

- Uses workflow analyses to examine current practice, workflow, and the potential impact of an informatics solution on that workflow.

- Conducts a needs analysis to refine the issue or problem when necessary.

- Involves the healthcare consumer, family, interprofessional team, and key stakeholders, as appropriate, in relevant data collection.

- Prioritizes data collection activities.

- Uses analytical models, algorithms, and tools that facilitate assessment. One example of an assessment algorithm is PIECES:

  - **P**erformance—throughput or response time;

  - **I**nformation—outputs, inputs, and/or stored data;

  - **E**conomics—costs versus profits;

  - **C**ontrol—too little security or control or too much control or security;

  - **E**fficiency—people, machines, or computers waste time, and;

  - **S**ervice—inaccurate, inconsistent, unreliable, hard to learn, difficult to use, inflexible, incompatible, not coordinated with other systems (Wetherbe, 1994).

- Synthesizes available data, information, evidence, and knowledge relevant to the situation to identify patterns and variances.

- Applies ethical, legal, and privacy regulations and policies for the collection, maintenance, use, and dissemination of data and information.

- Documents relevant data in a retrievable format.

Standard 2. Diagnosis, Problems, and Issues Identification

The informatics nurse analyzes assessment data to identify diagnoses, problems, issues, and opportunities for improvement.

COMPETENCIES

The informatics nurse:

- Derives diagnoses, problems, needs, issues, and opportunities for improvement based on assessment data.

- Validates the diagnoses, problems, needs, issues, and opportunities for improvement with the healthcare consumer, family, interprofessional team, and key stakeholders when possible and appropriate.

- Identifies actual or potential risks to the healthcare consumer's health and safety, or barriers to health, which may include, but are not limited to, interpersonal, systematic, or environmental circumstances.

- Uses standardized clinical terminologies, taxonomies, and decision support tools, when available, to identify problems, needs, issues, and opportunities for improvement.

- Documents problems, needs, issues, and opportunities for improvement in a manner that facilitates the discovery of expected outcomes and development of a plan.

Standard 3. Outcomes Identification

The informatics nurse identifies expected outcomes for a plan individualized to the healthcare consumer or the situation.

COMPETENCIES

The informatics nurse:

- Involves the healthcare consumer, family, healthcare providers, and key stakeholders in formulating expected outcomes when possible and appropriate.

- Defines expected outcomes in terms of the healthcare consumer, healthcare worker, and other stakeholders; their values; ethical considerations; and environmental, organizational, or situational considerations.

- Formulates expected outcomes after considering associated risks, benefits, costs, available expertise, evidence-based knowledge, and environmental factors.

- Develops expected outcomes that provide direction for project team members, the healthcare team, and key stakeholders.

- Includes a time estimate for the attainment of expected outcomes.

- Modifies expected outcomes based on changes in the status or evaluation of the situation.

- Documents expected outcomes as measurable goals.

**ADDITIONAL COMPETENCIES FOR THE
INFORMATICS NURSE SPECIALIST**

The informatics nurse specialist:

- Identifies expected outcomes that incorporate scientific evidence and are achievable through implementation of evidence-based practices.

- Identifies expected outcomes that maximize quality, efficiency, and effectiveness balanced with economy.

- Differentiates outcomes requiring care process interventions from those requiring system-level interventions.

- Supports the use and integration of clinical guidelines into practice, information management system solutions, and knowledge bases.

Standard 4. Planning

The informatics nurse develops a plan that prescribes strategies, alternatives, and recommendations to attain expected outcomes.

COMPETENCIES

The informatics nurse:

- Develops a customized plan considering clinical and business characteristics of the environment and situation.

- Develops the plan in collaboration with the healthcare consumer, family, healthcare team, key stakeholders, and others, as appropriate.

- Establishes the plan priorities with key stakeholders and others as appropriate.

- Incorporates strategies in the plan to address each of the identified diagnoses, problems, needs, and issues.

- Incorporates planned strategies addressing health and wholeness across the life span.

- Incorporates an implementation pathway or timeline within the plan.

- Considers the clinical, financial, social, and economic impact of the plan on the stakeholders.

- Integrates current scientific evidence, trends, and research into the planning process.

- Utilizes the plan to provide direction for the healthcare team and other stakeholders.

- Integrates current statutes, rules and regulations, and standards within the planning process and plan.

- Modifies the plan according to the ongoing assessment of the healthcare consumer's response and other outcome indicators.

- Integrates informatics principles in the design of interprofessional processes to address identified situations or issues.

- Documents the plan in a manner that uses standardized terminologies and taxonomies.

Standard 5. Implementation

The informatics nurse implements the identified plan.

COMPETENCIES

The informatics nurse:

■ Partners with the healthcare consumer, healthcare team, and others, as appropriate, to implement the plan on time, within budget, and within plan requirements.

■ Utilizes health information technology to measure, record, and retrieve healthcare consumer data, implement and support the nursing process, and improve overall healthcare outcomes.

■ Uses specific evidence-based actions and processes to resolve diagnoses, problems, or issues to achieve the defined outcomes.

■ Advocates for health care that is sensitive to the needs of healthcare consumers, with emphasis on the needs of diverse populations and use of self-care theory.

■ Applies available healthcare technologies to maximize access and optimize outcomes for healthcare consumers.

■ Uses community and organizational resources systematically to implement the plan.

■ Collaborates with the healthcare team and other stakeholders from diverse backgrounds to implement and integrate the plan.

■ Accommodates different styles of communication used by healthcare consumers, families, healthcare providers, and others.

■ Implements the plan using principles and concepts of enterprise management, project management, and systems change theory.

■ Promotes the healthcare consumer's capacity for the optimal level of participation and problem-solving.

■ Fosters an organizational culture that supports implementation of the plan.

■ Incorporates new information and strategies to initiate change if desired outcomes are not achieved.

- Documents implementation and any modifications, including changes or omissions, of the identified plan.

ADDITIONAL COMPETENCIES FOR THE INFORMATICS NURSE SPECIALIST

The informatics nurse specialist:

- Facilitates utilization of systems, organizations, and community resources to implement the plan.

- Supports collaboration with nursing and other colleagues to implement the plan.

- Uses advanced communication skills to promote relationships between healthcare teams and healthcare consumers by providing open discussion of shared experiences using information technologies.

Standard 5a. Coordination of Activities

The informatics nurse coordinates planned activities.

COMPETENCIES

The informatics nurse:

- Organizes the components of the plan.

- Coordinates the implementation of the plan, including activities and resources necessary to achieve desired outcomes.

- Synthesizes data and information to prescribe necessary system and environmental support measures.

- Documents the coordination of delivery activities to have a successful implementation.

ADDITIONAL COMPETENCIES FOR THE INFORMATICS NURSE SPECIALIST

The informatics nurse specialist:

- Provides leadership in the coordination of information technology and healthcare activities for integrated delivery of efficient and cost-effective healthcare services.

- Coordinates system and community resources that enhance delivery of health care across continuums.

Standard 5b. Health Teaching and Health Promotion

The informatics nurse employs informatics solutions and strategies for education and teaching to promote health and a safe environment.

COMPETENCIES

The informatics nurse:

- Integrates informatics solutions, resources, ergonomics, and disability adaptations into clinical practice workflow and patient care routines.

- Applies technology to support the dissemination of evidence-based information to promote healthy lifestyle choices, risk reduction behaviors, disability and developmental adaptations, and preventive self-care.

- Introduces technology to facilitate healthcare consumer, staff, community, and population learning.

- Seeks opportunities for feedback and evaluation of the effectiveness of the strategies used.

- Evaluates health information resources for accuracy, readability, and comprehensibility to help healthcare consumers, families, clinicians, staff, and others needing access to quality health information. An example is obtaining shared data through credible organizations (e.g., the Net Foundation [http://www.hon.ch/], HealthIT.gov Policy Researchers & Implementers [http://www.healthit.gov/policy-researchers-implementers], and Centers for Medicare & Medicaid E.H.R. Incentive Programs [http://www.cms.gov/Regulations-and-Guidance/Legislation/EHRIncentivePrograms/index.html]).

- Assists consumer alliances and advocacy groups in the proper utilization of technology to perform health promotion activities.

- Creates informatics solutions for feedback and evaluation of the effectiveness of the educational content and teaching strategies used for continuing education and professional development programs.

Standard 5c. Consultation

The informatics nurse provides consultation to influence the identified plan, enhance the abilities of others, and effect change.

COMPETENCIES

The informatics nurse:

- Synthesizes data, information, knowledge, theoretical frameworks, and evidence when providing consultation.

- Facilitates the effectiveness of a consultation by involving healthcare consumers, healthcare team members, and stakeholders in decision-making processes.

- Communicates consultation recommendations that influence the identified plan, facilitate understanding by involved stakeholders, enhance the work of others, and effect change.

ADDITIONAL COMPETENCIES FOR THE INFORMATICS NURSE SPECIALIST

The informatics nurse specialist:

- Develops recommendations and strategies to address and resolve complex informatics issues and problems.

- Uses risk management techniques to mitigate risks and take advantage of opportunities.

- Establishes formal and informal consultative relationships that provide professional informatics development and mentorship opportunities.

- Promotes collaborative relationships for consultation with thought leaders to expand the influence of health information solutions in enhancing population health at local, regional, national, and international levels.

Standard 6. Evaluation

The informatics nurse evaluates progress toward attainment of outcomes.

COMPETENCIES

The informatics nurse:

- Conducts a systematic, ongoing, and criterion-based evaluation of the outcomes in relation to the structures and processes prescribed by the project plan and indicated timeline.

- Collaborates with the healthcare consumer, healthcare team members, and other key stakeholders involved in the plan or situation in the evaluation process.

- Evaluates, in partnership with the key stakeholders, the effectiveness of the planned strategies in relation to attainment of the expected outcomes.

- Evaluates the link between outcomes and evidence-based methods, tools, and guidelines.

- Evaluates the effectiveness of planned strategies in relation to attainment of the expected outcomes.

- Documents the results of the evaluation.

- Disseminates the results to key stakeholders and others involved, in accordance with organizational requirements and federal and state regulations.

ADDITIONAL COMPETENCIES FOR THE INFORMATICS NURSE SPECIALIST

The informatics nurse specialist:

- Synthesizes the results of the evaluation analyses to determine the impact of the plan on healthcare consumers, families, communities, resources, networks, and healthcare organizations.

- Uses the results of the evaluation analyses to make or recommend process or structural changes, including policy, procedure, or protocol development, as appropriate.

Standards of Professional Performance for Nursing Informatics

Standard 7. Ethics

The informatics nurse practices ethically.

COMPETENCIES

The informatics nurse:

- Uses *Code of Ethics for Nurses with Interpretive Statements* (ANA, 2001) to guide practice.

- Recognizes the centrality of the healthcare consumer and family as core members of any healthcare team.

- Uses nursing and informatics principles, standards, and methodologies in a manner that preserves and protects healthcare consumer autonomy, dignity, and rights.

- Employs informatics principles, standards, and methodologies to establish and maintain healthcare consumer confidentiality within legal and regulatory parameters.

- Evaluates factors related to privacy, security, and confidentiality in the use and handling of data, information, and knowledge.

- Contributes to resolving ethical issues involving healthcare consumers, colleagues, community groups, systems, and other stakeholders.

- Takes appropriate action regarding instances of illegal, unethical, or inappropriate behavior that could endanger or jeopardize the best interests of the healthcare consumer, others, or the organization.

- Reports illegal, incompetent, or impaired practices.

- Speaks up when appropriate to question healthcare practice when necessary for safety and quality improvement.

- Advocates for systems conducive to staff workflow.

- Advocates for healthcare consumer access to electronic healthcare records and mobile health technologies, and for the reduction of associated disparities.

- Seeks available resources as needed when formulating ethical decisions.

- Demonstrates a commitment to practicing self-care, managing stress, and connecting with self and others.

ADDITIONAL COMPETENCIES FOR THE INFORMATICS NURSE SPECIALIST

The informatics nurse specialist:

- Participates in interprofessional teams that address ethical risks, benefits, and outcomes.

- Informs administrators or others of the risks, benefits, and outcomes of programs and decisions that affect healthcare delivery.

- Promotes active engagement of stakeholders in the oversight and management of the exchange of data, information, and knowledge.

Standard 8. Education

The informatics nurse attains knowledge and competence that reflect current nursing and informatics practice.

COMPETENCIES
The informatics nurse:

- Participates in ongoing education to advance his or her knowledge base and professional practice.

- Demonstrates a commitment to lifelong learning through self-reflection and inquiry to address learning and personal growth needs.

- Seeks experiences that reflect current practice to maintain knowledge, skills, abilities, and judgment in informatics practice and role performance.

- Acquires knowledge and skills appropriate to the role, population, specialty area, setting, or situation.

- Seeks formal and independent learning experiences to develop and maintain professional skills and knowledge.

- Identifies individual learning needs based on nursing knowledge, nursing roles, and the changing needs of target populations.

- Participates in knowledge acquisition to support the evolution and continuous improvement of enterprise management in support of plan implementation.

- Participates in formal and informal consultations to address issues in nursing practice to improve education and knowledge bases, as well as to contribute evidence for best practice.

- Continues to examine and review clinical care issues and new practice modalities for implications related to informatics solutions and practice.

- Shares educational findings, experiences, and ideas with peers.

- Develops skills to contribute to a work environment conducive to the education of healthcare professionals.

- Promotes educational opportunities and programs related to informatics.

■ Contributes to educational opportunities and programs related to informatics.

■ Maintains professional records that provide evidence of competence and lifelong learning.

ADDITIONAL COMPETENCIES FOR THE INFORMATICS NURSE SPECIALIST

The informatics nurse specialist:

■ Uses current research findings and other evidence to expand knowledge, skills, abilities, and judgment; to enhance role performance; and to increase knowledge of professional issues.

■ Creates educational opportunities and programs related to informatics.

Standard 9. Evidence-Based Practice and Research

The informatics nurse integrates evidence and research findings into practice.

COMPETENCIES

The informatics nurse:

- Uses data to communicate evidence to promote effective care processes and decisions.

- Utilizes current evidence-based nursing knowledge, including research findings, to guide practice.

- Incorporates current evidence when initiating changes in nursing practice.

- Participates in the formulation of evidence-based practice as appropriate to her or his education level, background, and position.

- Shares personal or third-party research findings with colleagues and peers.

- Uses the skills and tools available to the informatics nurse for research studies.

ADDITIONAL COMPETENCIES FOR THE
INFORMATICS NURSE SPECIALIST

The informatics nurse specialist:

- Supports nursing knowledge by conducting or synthesizing research and other evidence to promote the discovery, examination, and evaluation of current practice, knowledge, theories, criteria, and creative approaches to improve healthcare outcomes.

- Promotes a climate of research and clinical inquiry.

- Promotes the efficient, effective, and secure use of electronic health record data.

- Identifies and promotes documentation standards that facilitate the development of clinical databases that will allow research (e.g., standard data sets and formatting of reports).

- Formally disseminates research findings through activities such as presentations, publications, consultation, and journal clubs.

Standard 10. Quality of Practice

The informatics nurse contributes to quality and effectiveness of nursing and informatics practice.

COMPETENCIES

The informatics nurse:

- Demonstrates quality by documenting the application of the nursing process in a responsible, accountable, and ethical manner, and by facilitating a unified or defined level of documentation by nurses in clinical practice.

- Uses the results of quality improvement activities to initiate changes in nursing and informatics practice and in the healthcare delivery system.

- Contributes to the development and continuous improvement of organizational systems that support the planning process.

- Uses creativity and innovation to enhance nursing and informatics practice to improve care delivery and client satisfaction, and reduce healthcare costs.

- Uses nursing informatics principles to utilize electronic health record data to analyze outcomes of nursing practice.

- Incorporates new knowledge to initiate changes in nursing and informatics practice if desired outcomes are not achieved.

- Uses informatics principles to participate in quality improvement. Activities may include:

  - Identifying aspects of practice important for quality monitoring.

  - Using appropriate indicators to monitor quality and effectiveness of nursing and informatics practice.

  - Collecting data to monitor quality and effectiveness of nursing and informatics practice.

  - Analyzing quality data to identify opportunities to improve nursing and informatics practice.

  - Formulating recommendations to improve nursing and informatics practice or outcomes.

  - Implementing activities to enhance the quality of nursing and informatics practice.

■ Developing, implementing, and/or evaluating policies, procedures, and guidelines to improve the quality of practice.

■ Participating on and/or leading interprofessional teams to evaluate clinical care or health services.

■ Participating in and/or leading efforts to minimize costs and unnecessary duplication.

■ Integrating human–computer interaction (HCI) principles to improve nursing workflow, delivery of care, and client access to health information.

■ Analyzing factors to improve quality, user and client safety, and effectiveness.

■ Analyzing organizational systems for barriers to quality healthcare consumer outcomes.

■ Implementing processes to remove or weaken barriers within organizational systems.

ADDITIONAL COMPETENCIES FOR THE INFORMATICS NURSE SPECIALIST

The informatics nurse specialist:

■ Provides leadership in the design and implementation of quality improvements.

■ Designs innovations in data collection and management to effect change in practice and improve health outcomes.

■ Evaluates the practice environment and quality of nursing care rendered in relation to existing evidence.

■ Identifies opportunities for the generation and use of research and evidence.

■ Obtains and maintains professional informatics certification.

■ Uses the results of quality improvement studies to initiate changes in nursing practice and the healthcare delivery system.

■ Promotes the ability of nursing personnel to use electronic documentation systems to effectively describe the nursing process.

Standard 11. Communication

The informatics nurse communicates effectively in a variety of formats in all areas of practice.

COMPETENCIES

The informatics nurse:

- Assesses communication preferences of healthcare consumers, families, and colleagues.

- Supports communication preferences of healthcare consumers, families, and colleagues.

- Assesses her or his own communication skills in encounters with healthcare consumers, families, and colleagues to identify gaps, areas for improvement, and opportunities for education.

- Seeks continuous improvement of communication skills and technologies.

- Seeks continuous improvement of conflict resolution skills.

- Conveys information to healthcare consumers, families, the interprofessional team, and others using communication formats that promote accuracy and accessibility.

- Communicates strategies to improve and enhance the value of documentation.

- Problem-solves to report, address, and resolve hazards and errors in care or the practice environment.

- Identifies strategies and technologies to enhance communication among healthcare clinicians and consumers to minimize risks, especially those associated with transitions in care.

- Contributes the informatics professional perspective in discussions with the interprofessional team.

Standard 12. Leadership

The informatics nurse demonstrates leadership in the professional practice setting and the profession.

COMPETENCIES

The informatics nurse:

- Promotes the organization's vision, the associated goals, and the strategic plan.

- Demonstrates a commitment to continuous education and lifelong learning for self and others, especially related to informatics content.

- Mentors colleagues for the advancement of nursing informatics practice, the profession, and quality health care.

- Treats colleagues with respect, trust, and dignity.*

- Demonstrates advanced communication and conflict resolution skills.

- Participates in professional and informatics organizations.

- Seeks ways to advance nursing autonomy and accountability.*

- Influences the development and implementation of healthcare policy involving healthcare consumers and the profession.

ADDITIONAL COMPETENCIES FOR THE INFORMATICS NURSE SPECIALIST

The informatics nurse specialist:

- Influences decision-making bodies to improve the professional practice environment and healthcare consumer outcomes.

- Provides direction to enhance the effectiveness of the interprofessional team.

- Promotes and develops nursing informatics by interpreting its role for healthcare consumers, families, and others.

---

* Board of Higher Education & Massachusetts Organization of Nurse Executives [BHE/MONE], 2006.

- Models expert nursing informatics practice to interprofessional team members and healthcare consumers.

- Mentors colleagues in the acquisition of clinical knowledge, skills, abilities, and judgment.

- Promotes the use of data, information, knowledge, and wisdom to improve healthcare delivery and support effective nursing practice.

- Identifies opportunities to share innovative practice.

Standard 13. Collaboration

The informatics nurse collaborates with the healthcare consumer, family, and others in the conduct of nursing and informatics practice.

COMPETENCIES

The informatics nurse:

■ Partners with others to effect change and produce positive outcomes through the sharing of data, information, and knowledge of the healthcare consumer and/or situation.

■ Communicates with the healthcare consumer, family, and others regarding provision of care and the role of technology in that care.

■ Implements strategies to increase healthcare consumer use of personal health records (PHRs) and similar health information technology (IT) tools to engage more fully in their health and health care.

■ Implements strategies to increase healthcare consumers' participation and ownership in their care process and to take greater ownership of their own outcomes and safety in all healthcare venues.

■ Participates in building consensus or resolving conflict in the context of patient care and the application of technology to support that care.

■ Applies group process and negotiation techniques with healthcare consumers and colleagues.

■ Adheres to standards and applicable codes of conduct that govern behavior among peers and colleagues to create a work environment that promotes cooperation, respect, and trust.

■ Promotes the development and use of electronic health records that are focused on patient-centered outcomes and decision-making.

■ Engages in teamwork and team-building processes.

ADDITIONAL COMPETENCIES FOR THE INFORMATICS NURSE SPECIALIST

The informatics nurse specialist:

- Partners with others, within and outside of health care, to enhance healthcare consumer outcomes through interprofessional activities, such as education, consultation, management, technological development, or research opportunities to create technologies that support consumer engagement.

- Invites the contribution of the healthcare consumer, family, and team members in order to achieve optimal outcomes.

- Leads in establishing, improving, and sustaining collaborative relationships to design and implement technologies to achieve safe, quality health care.

Standard 14. Professional Practice Evaluation

The informatics nurse evaluates his or her own nursing practice in relation to professional practice standards and guidelines, relevant statutes, rules, and regulations.

COMPETENCIES

The informatics nurse:

- Supports delivery of appropriate care and services in a culturally, ethnically, and developmentally sensitive manner.

- Engages in self-evaluation of practice on a regular basis, identifying areas of strength as well as areas in which professional growth would be beneficial.

- Obtains informal feedback regarding her or his own practice from health-care consumers, peers, professional colleagues, and others.

- Participates in peer review as appropriate.

- Takes action to achieve goals identified during the evaluation process.

- Provides the evidence for practice decisions and actions as part of the informal and formal evaluation processes.

- Interacts with peers and colleagues to enhance his or her own professional nursing practice or role performance.

- Provides peers with formal or informal constructive feedback regarding their practice or role performance.

ADDITIONAL COMPETENCIES FOR THE INFORMATICS NURSE SPECIALIST

The informatics nurse specialist:

- Engages in a formal process seeking feedback regarding her or his own practice from healthcare consumers, peers, professional colleagues, and others.

- Provides mentorship to informatics nurses and those studying to become informatics nurses.

Standard 15. Resource Utilization

The informatics nurse employs appropriate resources to plan and implement informatics and associated services that are safe, effective, and fiscally responsible.

COMPETENCIES

The informatics nurse:

- Monitors the healthcare information needs of individual consumers and communities, as well as the available operational and technical enterprise resources to achieve desired outcomes.

- Identifies opportunities, potential for harm/risk, complexity of the task, and desired outcomes when considering resource allocation.

- Identifies best practices and evidence for safety and care outcomes when evaluating the allocation of resources.

- Supports the integration of clinical, human, financial, and technical resources to enhance and facilitate the healthcare decision-making process.

- Advocates for resources, including technology, that enhance nursing practice.

- Modifies practice as technologies and resources emerge and evolve.

- Assists the healthcare consumer and family in researching and securing appropriate and affordable information and technology resources to address care needs across the healthcare continuum.

ADDITIONAL COMPETENCIES FOR THE INFORMATICS NURSE SPECIALIST

The informatics nurse specialist:

- Uses organizational and community resources and information technologies to empower the interprofessional team and enhance planning initiatives.

- Formulates solutions that address the requirements of informatics projects, such as project plan, software specification documents, and request for proposal (RFP).

- Designs evaluation strategies that measure fiscal outcomes, user satisfaction, and project effectiveness.

Standard 16. Environmental Health

The informatics nurse supports practice in a safe and healthy environment.

COMPETENCIES

The informatics nurse:

- Attains knowledge of environmental health concepts, such as implementation of environmental health strategies.

- Promotes a practice environment that reduces ergonomic and environmental health risks for workers and healthcare consumers.

- Assesses the practice environment for factors that threaten health, such as sound, odor, noise, electromagnetic forces, and light.

- Advocates for the judicious and appropriate use of ergonomic and environmentally safe products in health care.

- Communicates environmental health risks and exposure reduction strategies to healthcare consumers, families, colleagues, and communities.

- Employs scientific evidence to determine if a product or treatment is an environmental or ergonomic risk.

- Participates in strategies to promote healthy communities.

- Assists in the development of health and safety alerts within the clinical documentation and technology solutions.

- Advocates for convenient electronic resources that allow quick and easy access to information.

ADDITIONAL COMPETENCIES FOR THE INFORMATICS NURSE SPECIALIST

The informatics nurse specialist:

- Creates partnerships that promote sustainable environmental health policies and conditions.

- Analyzes the impact of social, political, and economic influences on the environment and human health exposures.

- Critically evaluates the manner in which environmental health issues are presented by the popular media.

- Advocates for implementation of environmental principles in nursing practice.

- Supports nurses in advocating for and implementing environmental principles in nursing practice.

Glossary

Data. Discrete entities that are described objectively without interpretation.

Human–computer interaction (HCI). The study of how people design, implement, and evaluate interactive computer systems in the context of users' tasks and work (Nelson & Staggers, 2014, pp. 511–512).

Informatics nurse (IN). A registered nurse with an interest or experience in an informatics field, most often identified as nursing informatics.

Informatics nurse specialist (INS). A registered nurse with formal, graduate-level education in informatics or a related field.

Information. Data that are interpreted, organized, or structured.

Knowledge. Information that is synthesized so that relationships are identified and formalized.

Meaningful use. Delineated sets of specific objectives associated with purchase and use of health information technology solutions and quality reporting that must be met to qualify for federal incentive payments.

Metadata. Data about data. Metadata describes how, when, and by whom a particular set of data was collected, and how the data are formatted (http://www.webopedia.com/TERM/M/metadata.html).

Operational architecture. A data management process that enables a responsive end-to-end healthcare information environment in which: (1) information exchange processes are transparent and actionable; (2) the means to produce, exchange, and use information are protected; and (3) resources are allocated based on operational requirements and implemented through the use of precedence, priority, and resource allocation techniques.

System life cycle. Conceptual model or framework used to formally describe each stage of a living or nonliving system, such as an information system.

Usability. Extent to which a product can be used by specific users in a specific context to achieve specific goals with effectiveness, efficiency, and satisfaction.

Wisdom. The appropriate use of knowledge to manage and solve human problems.

References

Agency for Toxic Substances & Disease Registry. (2010). *Environmental health nursing initiative.* Retrieved from http://www.atsdr.cdc.gov/EHN/

American Association of Colleges of Nursing (AACN). (2006). *The essentials of doctoral education for advanced nursing practice.* Retrieved from http://www.aacn.nche.edu/publications/position/DNPEssentials.pdf

American Association of Colleges of Nursing (AACN). (2008). *The essentials of baccalaureate education for professional nursing practice.* Retrieved from http://www.aacn.nche.edu/education-resources/baccessentials08.pdf

American Association of Colleges of Nursing (AACN). (2011). *The essentials of master's education in nursing.* Retrieved from http://www.aacn.nche.edu/education-resources/MastersEssentials11.pdf

American Association of Colleges of Nursing (AACN). (2013). *QSEN informatics initiative: Background & overview.* Retrieved from http://www.aacn.nche.edu/qsen-informatics/background overview

American Association of Colleges of Nursing (AACN). (2014). Key differences between DNP and PhD/DNS programs. Retrieved from http://www.aacn.nche.edu/dnp/ContrastGrid.pdf

American Nurses Association (ANA). (2001*). Code of ethics for nurses with interpretive statements.* Silver Spring, MD: Nursesbooks.org.

American Nurses Association (ANA). (2010). *Nursing: Scope and standards of practice* (2nd ed.). Silver Spring, MD: Nursesbooks.org.

American Nurses Association (ANA). (2012, June 4). ANA recognized terminologies that support nursing practice. Retrieved from http://www.nursingworld.org/MainMenuCategories/ThePracticeofProfessionalNursing/NursingStandards/Recognized-Nursing-Practice-Terminologies.pdf

American Nurses Association (ANA) & International Society of Nurses in Genetics (ISONG). (2011). *Essential genetic and genomic competencies for nurses with graduate degrees.* http://www.nursingworld.org/MainMenuCategories/EthicsStandards/Genetics-1/ANA-and-ISONG-Announce-New-Publication.html

American Nurses Credentialing Center (ANCC). (2013). *2013 role delineation study: Nursing informatics—National survey results.* Retrieved from http://www.nursecredentialing.org/Certification/NurseSpecialties/Informatics/RELATED-LINKS/Informatics-2013RDS.pdf

American Organization of Nurse Executives. (2005). *The AONE nurse executive competencies.* Retrieved from http://www.aone.org/resources/leadership%20tools/PDFs/AONE_NEC.pdf

American Organization of Nurse Executives (AONE). (2012). *Position paper: Nursing informatics executive leader.* Retrieved from http://www.aone.org/resources/leadership%20tools/PDFs/AONE_Technology_Committee_CNIO_Position_Paper.pdf

American Telemedicine Association (ATA). (n.d.). *What is telemedicine?* Retrieved from http://www.americantelemed.org/about-telemedicine/what-is-telemedicine#.U7m7n7GmU1I

American Telemedicine Association (ATA). (2013). *Standards and guidelines.* Retrieved from http://www.healthit.gov/providers-professionals/community-college-consortia

Ash, J. S., Berg, M., & Coiera, E. (2004). Some unintended consequences of information technology in health care: The nature of patient care information system-related errors. *Journal of American Medical Informatics Association, 11*(2), 104–112. doi:10.1197/jamia.M1471

Ash, J. S., Sittig, D. F., Dykstra, R., Campbell, E., & Guappone, K. (2009). The unintended consequences of computerized provider order entry: Findings from a mixed methods exploration. *International Journal of Medical Informatics, 78*(suppl. 1), S69–S76. doi:10.1016/jmedinf.2008.07.015

Baer, A., Rodriguez, C. V., & Duchin, J. S. (2011). An automated system for public health surveillance of school absenteeism. *Journal of Public Health Management Practice, 17*, 59–64.

Bassendowski, S. (2013). Holograms in healthcare [Technology in Education column]. *Canadian Journal of Nursing Informatics, 8*(3). Retrieved from http://cjni.net/journal/?p=3256

Benner, P. E. (1984). *Novice to expert: Excellence and power in clinical nursing practice.* Reading, MA: Addison Wesley.

Benner, P. E., Hooper-Kyriakidis, P. L., & Stannard, D. (2011). *Clinical wisdom and interventions in acute and critical care: A thinking-in-action approach.* New York, NY: Springer.

Blum, B. (1986). *Clinical information systems.* New York, NY: Springer-Verlag.

Board of Higher Education & Massachusetts Organization of Nurse Executives (BHE/MONE). (2006). *Creativity and connections: Building the framework for the future of nursing education. Report from the Invitational Working Session, March 23-24, 2006.* Burlington, MA: MONE. Retrieved from www. mass.edu/currentinit/documents/NursingCreativityAndConnections.pdf

Brame, C. (2013). Flipping the classroom. Retrieved from http://cft. vanderbilt.edu/guides-sub-pages/flipping-the-classroom/

Calzone, K., et al. (Genomic Nursing State of the Science Advisory Panel). (2013). A blueprint for genomic nursing science. *Journal of Nursing Scholarship, 45*(1), 1 9. Retrieved from http://www.ninr.nih.gov/sites/www. ninr.nih.gov/files/jnu_12007_Rev_EV.pdf

Carroll, R., & Nakamura, P. (2011). *Risk management handbook for healthcare organizations, volume 1: The essentials.* San Francisco, CA: Jossey-Bass.

Chang, J., Poynton, M. R., Gassert, C. A., & Staggers, N. (2011). Nursing informatics competencies required of nurses in Taiwan. *International Journal of Medical Informatics, 80*(5), 332–340. doi:http://dx.doi. org/10.1016/j.ijmedinf.2011.01.011

Cho, I., Staggers, N., & Park, I. (2010). Nurses' responses to differing amounts and information content in a diagnostic computer-based decision support application. *CIN: Computers, Informatics, Nursing, 28*(2), 95–102.

Choi, J. (2012). Comparative assessment of informatics competencies in three undergraduate programs. *Online Journal of Nursing Informatics, 6*(2). http://ojni.org/issues/?p=1700

Choi, J., & Bakken, S. (2013). Validation of the Self-Assessment of Nursing Informatics Competencies Scale among undergraduate and graduate nursing students. *Journal of Nursing Education, 52*(5), 275–282. doi:10.3928/01484834-20130412-01

CHPS®. (2014). Certified in healthcare privacy and security. Retrieved from http://www.ahima.org/certification/chps

CHTS. (2013). Certified healthcare technology specialist. Retrieved from http://www.ahima.org/certification/chts

Community College Consortia. (n.d.). Participating community colleges. Retrieved from http://www.healthit.gov/providers-professionals/participating-community-colleges

Community Health Nurses' Initiatives Group. (2013). Retrieved from http://www.chnig.org/

Cronenwett, L., Sherwood, G., Barnsteiner, J., Disch, J., Johnson, J., Mitchell, P., & Warren, J. (2007). Quality and safety education for nurses. *Nursing Outlook, 55*(3), 122–131.

Duke University. (2012). DNP-PhD comparison. Retrieved from http://nursing.duke.edu/academics/programs/dnp/dnp-phd-comparison

Emory University. (2011, September 16). University-industry partnerships drive economic impact, improvements in health care. Retrieved from http://shared.web.emory.edu/whsc/news/releases/2011/09/university-industry-partnerships-drive-economic-impact,-improvements-in-health-care.html

Englebardt, S., & Nelson, R. (2002). *Health care informatics: An interdisciplinary approach.* St. Louis, MO: Mosby-Year Book.

e-Patients.net. (2013). Retrieved from http://e-patients.net/

Feather, J., & Sturges, P. (Eds.). *The international encyclopedia of information and library science* (2nd ed.), s.v. "Information management" 263–278. London, UK: Routledge, 2002. Retrieved from http://informationr.net/tdw/publ/papers/encyclopedia_entry.html

Flood, L. S., Gasiewicz, N., & Delpier, T. (2010). Integrating information literacy across a BSN curriculum. *Journal of Nursing Education, 49*(2), 101–104. doi:10.3928/01484834-20091023-01

Graves, J., & Corcoran, S. (1989). The study of nursing informatics. *Image, 21*(4), 227–230.

Guo, J., Irdbarren, S., Kapsandoy, S., Perri, S., & Staggers, N. (2011). eMAR user interfaces: A call for ubiquitous usability evaluations and product redesign. *Applied Clinical Informatics, 2*(2), 202–204.

Health Information and Management Systems Society (HIMSS). (2014). *2014 nursing informatics workforce survey.* Chicago, IL: Author.

Health Resources and Services Administration (HRSA). (n.d.). Telehealth. Retrieved from http://www.hrsa.gov/ruralhealth/about/telehealth/

Healthcare Leadership Alliance (HLA). (2005). *HLA competency directory, 2.0.* Retrieved from http://www.healthcareleadershipalliance.org/

Healthcare Leadership Alliance (HLA). (2013). Introducing the HLA Competency Directory, version 2.0. Retrieved from http://www.healthcareleadershipalliance.org/directory.htm

HealthIT.gov. (n.d.). *Connecting health and care for the nation: A 10-year vision to achieve an interoperable health IT infrastructure.* Retrieved from http://www.healthit.gov/sites/default/files/ONC10yearInteroperabilityConceptPaper.pdf

HealthIT.gov (2009.). *HITECH Act.* Retrieved from http://www.hhs.gov/ocr/privacy/hipaa/understanding/coveredentities/hitechact.pdf

HealthIT.gov (2013.). Health IT curriculum resources for educators. Retrieved from http://www.healthit.gov/providers-professionals/health-it-curriculum-resources-educators

HealthIT.gov. (2014). *Competency examination program.* Retrieved from http://www.healthit.gov/providers-professionals/competency-examination-program

HealthIT Help Center Workforce Programs. (n.d.). *Workforce programs.* Retrieved from http://www.healthit.gov/providers-professionals/workforce-development-programs

Hebda, T., & Calderone, T. (2010). What nurse educators need to know about the TIGER initiative. *Nurse Educator, 35*(2), 56–60.

Hemmerly-Brown, A. (2011). DoD gives PTSD help "second life" in virtual reality. Retrieved from http://www.army.mil/article/50751/dod-gives-ptsd-help-second-life-in-virtual-reality/

Hinman, A. R., & Ross, D. A. (2010, April). Immunization registries can be building blocks for national health information. *Health Affairs, 29*(4), 676–682. doi:http://dx.doi.org/10.1377/hlthaff.2007.0594

Hodges, L. & Wierz, C. (2012). *The emerging role of the chief nursing information officer: What is the current state?* (Presented at HIMSS12 Nursing Informatics Symposium, Feb. 20.) Healthcare Information and Management Systems Society: Chicago. Retrieved from http://69.59.162.218/HIMSS2012/Venetian%20Sands%20Expo%20Center/2.20.12_Mon/Marcello%204404/Mon_1030/NI7-11_Chris_Wierz_Marcello%204404/NI7Wierz.pdf

Houlihan, P. (n.d.). *RIC researchers explore promising new robotic technology.* Retrieved from http://lifecenter.ric.org/index.php?tray=content&tid=top103&cid=6676

Hsu, C. E., Dunn, K., Juo, H.-H., Danko, R., Johnson, D., Mas, F. S., & Sheu, J.-J. (2012). Understanding public health informatics competencies for mid-tier public health practitioners: A web-based survey. *Health Informatics Journal, 18*(1), 66–76. doi:10.1177/1460458211424000

Huang, C., Chen, C., & Chung, H. (2005). Application of facial electromyography in computer mouse access for people with disabilities. *Disability and Rehabilitation, 28*(4), 231–237.

Institute of Medicine (IOM). (1999). *To err is human: Building a safer health system.* Washington, DC: National Academies Press.

Institute of Medicine (IOM). (2001). *Crossing the quality chasm: A new health system for the 21st century.* Washington, DC: National Academies Press.

Institute of Medicine (IOM). (2010). *The future of nursing: Leading change, advancing health.* Washington, DC: National Academies Press.

Institute of Medicine (IOM) (2012). *Health IT and patient safety: Building safer systems for better care.* Washington, DC: National Academies Press.

International Council of Nurses (ICN). (2013). *ICNP®*. Retrieved from http://www.icn.ch/pillarsprograms/international-classification-for-nursing-practice-icnpr/

International Organization for Standardization (2009). *Ergonomics of human system interaction - Part 210: Human-centered design for interactive systems (formerly known as 13407)*. ISO FDIS 9241-210:2009

Interprofessional Education Collaborative Expert Panel. (2011). *Core competencies for interprofessional collaborative practice: Report of an expert panel*. Washington, D.C.: Interprofessional Education Collaborative. Retrieved from http://www.aacn.nche.edu/education-resources/ipecreport.pdf

Jain, K. K. (2008). Nanomedicine: Application of nanobiotechnology in medical practice. *Medical Principles and Practice. 17*(2):89–101. doi: 10.1159/000112961. Epub 2008 Feb 19. Retrieved from http://www.futuremedicine.com/doi/pdf/10.2217/nnm.09.12

Koppel, R., Metlay, J. P., Cohen, A., et al. (2005). Role of computerized physician order entry systems in facilitating medication errors. *Journal of the American Medical Association, 293*(10), 1197–1203. doi:10:1001/jama.293.10.1197

Leventhal, R. (2010, May 8). California hospitals to utilize robot technology to treat stroke patients. *Healthcare Informatics* Retrieved from http://www.healthcare-informatics.com/news-item/california-hospitals-utilize-robot-technology-treat-stroke-patients

Maojo, V., García-Remesal, M., Iglesia, D. D., Crespo, J., Pérez-Rey, D., Chiesa, S., & Kulikowski, C. A. (2011). Nanoinformatics: Developing advanced informatics applications for nanomedicine. *Fundamental Biomedical Technologies, 5*, 847–860. doi:10.1007/978-94-007-1248-5_26

McGonigle, D., Hunter, K. M., Hebda, T., & Hill, T. (2013). *Assessment of level 3 and level 4 nursing informatics (NI) competencies tool development*. Poster presented at the Summer Institute in Nursing Informatics (SINI), "Beyond Stage 7 and Meaningful Use: What's Next?"

McGonigle, D., & Mastrian, K. G. (2015). Emerging technologies and the generation of knowledge. In *Nursing informatics and the foundation of knowledge* (3rd ed., pp. 485–537). Burlington, MA: Jones & Bartlett Learning.

Michaelsen, L. K. (n.d.). Getting started with team-based learning. Retrieved from http://faculty.ucmo.edu/teambasedlearning/docs/Getting%20 Started%20with%20TBL.pdf

Morton, A. (2011, May 12). *UBT Program: Preparing the health IT leaders of tomorrow, today.* Retrieved from http://www.healthit. gov/buzz-blog/university-based-training/ubt-program-preparing-health-leaders-tomorrow-today/

National League for Nursing (NLN). (2008). Preparing the next generation of nurses to practice in a technology-rich environment: An informatics agenda. Retrieved from http://www.nln.org/aboutnln/ PositionStatements/informatics_052808.pdf

Nelson, R. (2002). Major theories supporting health care informatics. In: Englebardt, S., & Nelson, R., eds., *Health Care Informatics: An Interdisciplinary Approach.* St. Louis, MO: Mosby-Year Book, 3–2.7.

Nelson, R., & Joos, I. (1989). On language in nursing: From data to wisdom. *PLN Vision,* 6.

Nelson, R., & Staggers, N. (Eds.) (2014). *Health informatics: An interprofessional approach.* St. Louis, MO: Elsevier Mosby.

Nielscn, J. (2012, January 4). Usability 101: Introduction to usability. Retrieved from www.nngroup.com/articles/usability-101-introduction-to-usability

Public Health Informatics Institute (PHII). (2009). The value of health IT in improving population health and transforming public health practice. Retrieved from http://www.phii.org/resources/view/151/The%20 Value%20of%20Health%20IT%20in%20Improving%20Population%20 Health%20and%20Transforming%20Public%20Health%20Practice

QSEN Institute. (2012a). The evolution of the Quality and Safety Education for Nurses (QSEN) initiative. Retrieved from http://qsen.org/about-qsen/ project-overview/

QSEN Institute. (2012b). Graduate-level QSEN competencies, knowledge, skills and attitudes. Retrieved from http://www.aacn.nche.edu/faculty/ qsen/competencies.pdf

Registered Environmental Health Specialist Program. (2013). Retrieved from http://www.neha.org/credential/index.shtml#rehsrs_cred

Remus, S., & Kennedy, M. A. (2012). Innovation in transformative nursing leadership: Nursing informatics competencies and roles. *Canadian Journal of Nursing Leadership, 25*(4), 14–26.

Robotics Technology—Healthcare Robotics. (n.d.). Retrieved from http://www.robotxworld.com/channels/healthcare-robotics/

Scriven, M., & Paul, R. (1987). *Critical thinking as defined by the National Council for Excellence in Critical Thinking, 1987.* Presentation at the 8th Annual International Conference on Critical Thinking and Education Reform, Summer 1987. Retrieved from http://www.criticalthinking.org

Shadow Health. (2014). Physical Assessment [Digital Clinical Experience].Retrieved from http://www.shadowhealth.com/health-assessment.html.

Sibley, C. (2008). Web usability and aging. Retrieved from http://www.usability.gov/get-involved/blog/2008/12/aging-and-usability.html

Sittig, D. F., & Singh, H. (2010). A new sociotechnical model for studying health information technology in complex adaptive healthcare systems. *Quality & Safety in Heath Care, 19*, i68–i74.

Spector, N. (2013, May 9). *Description of NCSBN's Transition to Practice® (TTP) model.* Retrieved from https://www.ncsbn.org/13_TransitiontoPractice_modeldescription.pdf

Staggers, N. (2014). Improving the user experience for health information technology products. In R. Nelson & N. Staggers (Eds.), *Health informatics: An interdisciplinary approach* (pp. 337–350). St. Louis, MO: Elsevier.

Staggers, N., Gassert, C. A., & Curran, C. (2001). Informatics competencies for nurses at four levels of practice. *Journal of Nursing Education, 40*(7), 303–316.

Staggers, N., Gassert, C. A., & Curran, C. (2002). A Delphi study to determine informatics competencies for nurses at four levels of practice. *Nursing Research, 51*(6) 383–391.

Staggers, N., Jennings, B. M., & Lasome, C. E. (2010). A usability assessment of AHLTA in ambulatory clinics at a military medical center. *Military Medicine, 175*(7), 518–524.

Stead, W., & Lin, H. (2009). *Computational technology for effective health care: Immediate steps and strategic directions.* Washington, DC: National Academies Press.

Sternberger, C. S. (2012, March). Interactive learning environment: Engaging students using clickers. *Nursing Education Perspectives, 33*(2), 121–124. doi:http://dx.doi.org/10.5480/1536-5026-33.2.121

Technology Informatics Guiding Education Reform (TIGER). (2009). Informatics competencies for every practicing nurse: Recommendations from the TIGER collaborative. Retrieved from http://www. thetigerinitiative.org/docs/TigerReport_InformaticsCompetencies.pdf

ThinkGeek. (2014). Virtual keyboard. Retrieved from http://www.thinkgeek. com/brain/whereisit.cgi?t=virtual+keyboard

Topol, E. (2011). *The creative destruction of medicine: How the digital revolution will create better health care.* New York, NY: Perseus Books Group.

U.S. Food and Drug Administration (FDA) General Human Factors Information and Resource. Retrieved from http://www.fda.gov/ medicaldevices/deviceregulationandguidance/humanfactors/ucm124829. htm

Weiner, J. P., Kfuri, T., Chan, K., & Fowles, J. B. (2007, May–June). "e-iatrogenesis": The most critical unintended consequence of CPOE and other HIT. *Journal of the American Medical Informatics Association, 14*(3), 387–388; discussion 389.

Wisconsin Institute for Discovery. (n.d.). Living environments laboratory. Retrieved from http://wid.wisc.edu/research/lel/

World Health Organization (WHO). (2010). Framework for action on interprofessional education and collaborative practice. (WHO/HRH/ HPN/10.3) Geneva, Switzerland: Author. Retrieved from http:// whqlibdoc.who.int/hq/2010/WHO_HRH_HPN_10.3_eng.pdf?ua=1

Zhou, L. (2007). Natural language interface for information management on mobile devices. *Behaviour & Information Technology, 26*(3), 197–207.

Appendix A.

An Emerging Model of Wisdom

Susan Matney describes the development of wisdom through the use of knowledge in her model, Wisdom-in-Action for Clinical Nursing©. This model denotes that knowledge encompasses:

- The center core of clinical judgment;

- Values, relativism, and tolerance;

- Life span contextualism;

- Rich procedural knowledge; and

- Rich factual knowledge.

Antecedents to this knowledge are the person-related factors and the environmental factors of setting and systems. When nurses are put into a stressful situation that has a degree of uncertainty, their specialized knowledge mastery produces insight and intuition into the decision-making needed for action. This learning, reflection, and discovery of meaning for the situation become integrated into their inherent knowledge base or "wisdom" for future actions.

Figure 1. Matney Model of Wisdom-in-Action for Clinical Nursing©
(Work in progress; Permission to use granted by Susan Matney)

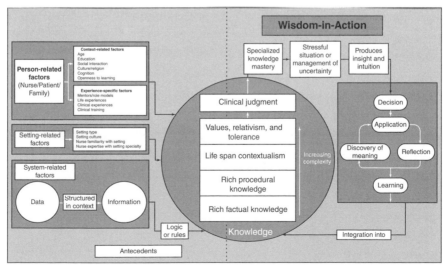

Appendix B.

Nursing Informatics: Scope and Standards of Practice (2008)

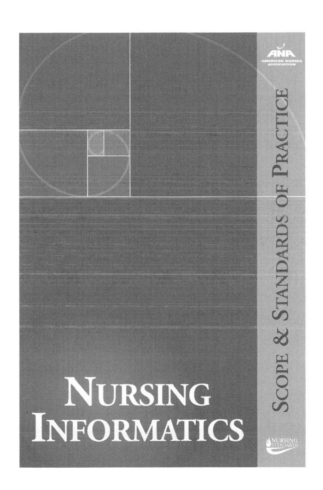

The content in this appendix is not current and is of historical significance only.

ACKNOWLEDGMENTS

Work Group Members (2007)

Nancy Staggers, PhD, RN, FAAN, Chairperson
Michele Calogero, MSN, RN
Margaret F. Budnik, DM, RN
Diane Castelli, RN
Melissa Christensen
Mary F. Clarke, PhD, RN, BC
Tina Dieckhaus, BSN, RN-BC, Leader, Integration and Tenets
Paulette Fraser, MS, RN-BC, Co-leader Metastructures
Josette Jones, PhD, RN-BC, Co-leader Competencies
Sally Kellum, MSN, RN-C
Rosemary Kennedy, MBA, RN, Co-leader NI Standards
Kathleen Krichbaum, RN, PhD
Sheryl LaCoursiere, PhD, RN-BC, Leader, Functional Areas
Angela Lewis, BSN, RN-BC
Teresa McCasky, MBA, BSN, RN-BC
Ramona Nelson, PhD, RN, FAAN, Co-leader, Metastructures
Agnes Padernal, PhD, RN
Amy Peck, RN
Mollie R. Poynton PhD, APRN
Loretta Schlachta-Fairchild, PhD, RN, CHE
Norma Street, MSN, RN
Sharon Sweeney Fee, PhD, RN, Leader, Ethics section
Dawn Weathersby, MS, RN, Co-leader NI Standards
Jill Winters, PhD, RN
Seth Wolpin PhD MPH RN, Co-leader Competencies
Lisa Wynn, MA, RN-BC

ANA Staff

Carol J. Bickford, PhD, RN-BC—Content editor
Yvonne D. Humes, MSA—Project coordinator
Therese Myers, JD—Legal counsel

The content in this appendix is not current and is of historical significance only.

CONTENTS

The content in this appendix is not current and is of historical significance only.

The content in this appendix is not current and is of historical significance only.

The content in this appendix is not current and is of historical significance only.

THE SCOPE OF NURSING INFORMATICS PRACTICE

Introduction

Nursing informatics (NI) is a specialty that integrates nursing science, computer science, and information science to manage and communicate data, information, knowledge, and wisdom in nursing practice. NI supports consumers, patients, nurses, and other providers in their decision-making in all roles and settings. This support is accomplished through the use of information structures, information processes, and information technology.

The goal of NI is to improve the health of populations, communities, families, and individuals by optimizing information management and communication. These activities include the design and use of informatics solutions and technology to support all areas of nursing, including, but not limited to, the direct provision of care, establishing effective administrative systems, designing useful decision support systems, managing and delivering educational experiences, enhancing lifelong learning, and supporting nursing research (Staggers & Thompson, 2002).

The NI definition remains essentially that found in *Scope and Standards of Nursing Informatics* (2001), but now includes the additional concept of wisdom. The term *individuals* refers to patients, healthcare consumers, and any other recipients of nursing care or informatics solutions. The term *patient* refers to consumers in both a wellness and illness model. The discussion of the definition and goal of nursing informatics evolved from work by Staggers and Thompson (2002).

Nursing informatics is one example of a discipline-specific informatics practice within the broader category of health informatics. NI has become well established within nursing since its recognition as a specialty for registered nurses by the American Nurses Association (ANA) in 1992. It focuses on the representation of nursing data, information, knowledge (Graves & Corcoran, 1989) and wisdom (Nelson & Loos, 1989; Englebardt & Nelson, 2002) as well as the management and communication of nursing information within the broader context of health informatics. Nursing informatics (per Brennan, 2002):

- provides a nursing perspective,

- illuminates nursing values and beliefs,

The content in this appendix is not current and is of historical significance only.

- denotes a practice base for nurses in nursing informatics,

- produces unique knowledge,

- distinguishes groups of practitioners,

- focuses on the phenomena of interest for nursing, and

- provides needed nursing language and word context to health informatics.

The scope and standards of practice address both informatics nurse specialists (INSs), those formally prepared at the graduate level in informatics or a related field, and informatics nurses (INs), generalists who have experience but are not educated at the graduate level. However, informatics practice is highly complex and in the near future all nurses working in this specialty will have studied at the graduate level.

Nursing Informatics: Scope and Standards of Practice expands on earlier work in NI, builds on historical knowledge (ANA, 1994, 1995, 2001), and includes new, state-of-the-art material for the specialty. Because of rapid changes in related sciences, NI roles, and advances in the science of informatics, a new document was needed. New material in this revision includes: a) the concept of wisdom in NI metastructures, b) redirecting the discussion of roles from job titles to functions that may be integrated into various NI roles and subspecializations, c) identifying commonalities between INSs and other informatics specialists, d) distinguishing between INs and INSs, e) expanding the coverage of NI competencies to describe typical NI competencies for typical NI functional areas, f) expanding the discussion of ethics, human-computer interaction, and the future of NI, g) integrating new functions across clinical practice and NI, and h) changing the section titled "Boundaries of Nursing Informatics" to a discussion of the cross-disciplinary nature of NI that acknowledges the blurred boundaries of other informatics and nursing specialties.

This revised scope and standards document serves in several functions:

- An outline of the attributes and definition of the specialty.

- A reference and guide for educators and NI practitioners.

- A reference for employers and regulatory agencies to assist with developing position descriptions, determining required informatics competencies, and initiating NI positions in health organizations.

- A source document for legal opinions, funding agencies, and others seeking to improve health through nursing informatics.

Metastructures, Concepts, and Tools of Nursing Informatics

To understand NI, first its metastructures, sciences, concepts, and tools should be explained. *Metastructures* are overarching concepts used in theory and science. Also of interest are the sciences underpinning NI, concepts and tools from information science and computer science, human–computer interaction and ergonomics concepts, and the phenomena of nursing.

Metastructures: Data, Information, Knowledge, and Wisdom

In the mid-1980s Blum (1986) introduced the concepts of data, information, and knowledge as a framework for understanding clinical information systems and their impact on health care. He classified the then current clinical information systems according to the three types of objects that these systems processed: data, information, and knowledge. He noted that the classification was artificial, with no clear boundaries, although it did represent a scale of increasing complexity. In 1989, Graves and Corcoran built on these ideas in their seminal study of nursing informatics using the concepts of data, information, and knowledge. They contributed two general principles to NI. The first was a definition of nursing informatics that has been widely accepted in the field. The second contribution of their 1989 contribution was an information model that identified data, information, and knowledge as key components of NI practice (Figure 1).

Drawing from Blum (1986), Graves and Corcoran defined the three concepts as follows:

- Data are discrete entities that are described objectively without interpretation.

- Information is data that are interpreted, organized, or structured.

- Knowledge is information that is synthesized so that relationships are identified and formalized.

Data, which are processed into information and then knowledge, may be obtained from individuals, families, communities, and populations.

The content in this appendix is not current and is of historical significance only.

Figure 1. Conceptual Framework for the Study of Nursing Knowledge.

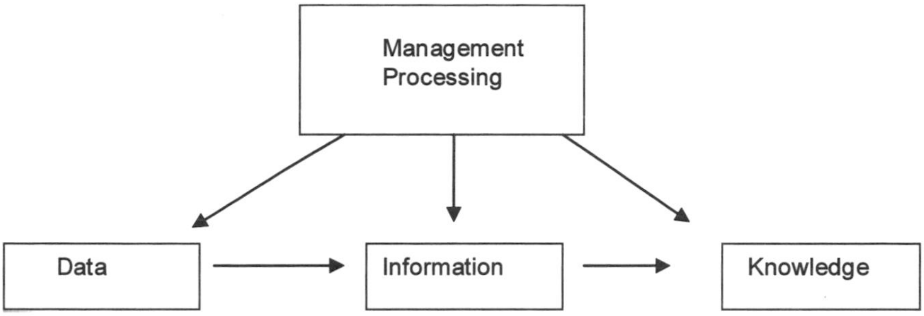

Source: Graves and Corcoran (1989) *Reprinted with permission of the publisher.*

Data, information, and knowledge are of value to nurses in all areas of practice. For example, data derived from direct care of an individual can then be compiled across persons and aggregated for decision-making by nurses, nurse administrators, or other health professionals. Further aggregation can encompass communities and populations. Nurse-educators can create case studies using these data, and nurse-researchers can access aggregated data for systematic study

The vital signs for an individual at a single moment—heart rate, respiration, temperature, and blood pressure—are an example of data. A chronological set of vital signs, placed into a context and used for longitudinal comparisons, is considered information. That is, a dropping blood pressure, increasing heart rate, respiratory rate, and fever in an elderly, catheterized person are recognized as abnormal. The recognition that the person may be septic and therefore may need certain nursing interventions reflects information synthesis (knowledge) based on nursing knowledge and experience.

Figure 2 builds on the work of Graves and Corcoran by depicting the relationship of data, information, knowledge, and a fourth level, wisdom. As data are transformed into information and information into knowledge, each level increases in complexity and requires greater application of human intellect. The X-axis represents interactions within and between the concepts as one moves from data to wisdom; the Y-axis represents the increasing complexity of the concepts and interrelationships.

The content in this appendix is not current and is of historical significance only.

Figure 2. The Relationship of Data, Information, Knowledge, and Wisdom

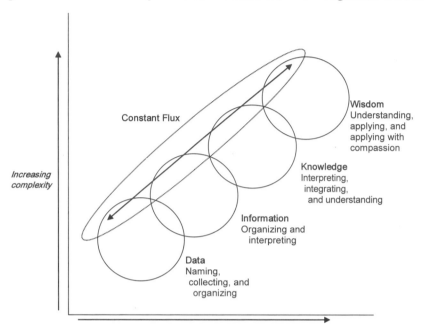

Reprinted with modification from Englebardt & Nelson, 2002, Figure 1-4, page 13 with permission from Elsevier.

Wisdom is defined as the appropriate use of knowledge to manage and solve human problems. It is knowing when and how to apply knowl- edge to deal with complex problems or specific human needs (Nelson, 1989; Englebardt & Nelson, 2002). While knowledge focuses on what is known, wis- dom focuses on the appropriate application of that knowledge. For ex- ample, a knowledge base may include several options for managing an anxious family, while wisdom would help decide which option is most appropriate for a specific family. The scope of NI is commensurate with the scope of nursing practice and nursing science, with a concentration on data, information, and knowledge. It is not limited by current tech- nologies. If NI were limited to what a computer can process, the disci- pline of informatics could not fully appreciate the relationships between nursing science and practice and information science and technology. Nursing informatics must take into consideration how nurses influence technology and how technology influences nursing. Understanding this

The content in this appendix is not current and is of historical significance only.

interaction makes it possible to understand how nurses create knowledge and how they use that knowledge in their practice.

The appropriate use of knowledge involves the integration of empirical, ethical, personal, and aesthetic knowledge into actions. The individual must apply a high level of empirical knowledge in understanding the current situation, apply a professional value system in considering possible actions, be able to predict the potential outcome of these actions with a high level of accuracy, and then have the will power to carry out the selected action in the given environment. An example of applied wisdom integrating these attributes in NI is the appropriate use of information management and technological tools to support effective nursing practice.

The addition of wisdom raises new and important research questions. It challenges the discipline to develop tools and processes for classifying, measuring, and encoding wisdom as it relates to nursing, NI, and informatics education. Research in these directions will help clarify the relationship between wisdom and the intuitive thinking of expert nurses. Such research will be invaluable in building information systems to support expert healthcare practitioners as well as support the less experienced in decision-making.

Two related forces are behind the expansion of the NI model to include wisdom. First, the initial work was limited to the types of objects processed by automated systems in the mid-1980s. However, NI is now concerned with the use of information technology to improve the access and quality of health care that is delivered to individuals, families, and communities. The addition of the concept of wisdom expands the model beyond technology and the processing of objects to include the interaction of the human with the technology and the resultant outcomes.

Second, nurses have been recognized as primary users and processors of information for over 40 years (Jydstrup & Gross, 1966; Zielstroff, 1981). Other authors have focused on the amount of time nurses actually spend administering direct care to patients or the time involved in documentation (Norrie, 1999; Jinks, 2000; Harrison, 2002). In fact, Jydstrup and Gross estimated in the 1960s that nurses in acute care spent 30% to 40% of their time in information processing activities. Hendrickson (1990) determined that nurses spent only 31% of their time

The content in this appendix is not current and is of historical significance only.

with patients. Other aspects of the nursing role included information management with ancillary services.

Sciences Underpinning Nursing Informatics

The work of Graves and Corcoran (1989) was a significant contribution to the NI definition of that was widely accepted in the field in the 1990s— that nursing informatics combines nursing science, information science, and computer science to manage and process nursing data, information, and knowledge to facilitate the delivery of health care. The central notion was that the application of these three core sciences was what made NI unique and differentiated it from other informatics specialties.

Other sciences may be required to solve informatics issues. Turley expanded the model of NI to include cognitive science (1996). Certainly the cognitive aspect of humans is a critical piece for INSs and INs to understand. However, other sciences may be equally critical. If the INS is implementing a system in an institution, for instance, an understanding of organizational theory may be germane (Staggers & Thompson, 2002). As science in general evolves, other sciences may emerge that need to be included in NI models.

Although the core sciences are foundational to the work in NI, the practice of the specialty can be considered an applied science rather than a basic science. The combination creates a unique blend that defines the NI specialty. Further, informatics realizes its full potential in health care when it is grounded in an established discipline; in this case, nursing. Computer and information science will have less impact applied in isolation and outside of a disciplinary framework.

Language as a Tool for Nursing Informatics

Many of the tools used by the informatics nurse and informatics nurse specialist are based on metastructures and concepts that incorporate knowledge from nursing and other health and information sciences. Nursing knowledge is refined by extracting, synthesizing, and analyzing data that defines nursing phenomena. The many different languages and ways of organizing data, information, and knowledge are built on nursing taxonomies and nomenclatures created over decades. ANA (2006a) has formalized these languages and vocabularies (listed in Table 1) after review by the Committee on Nursing Practice Information Infrastructure (CNPII).

The content in this appendix is not current and is of historical significance only.

Table 1. ANA Recognized Terminologies and Data Element Sets

	Setting Where Developed	Content
Data Element Sets		
NMDS Nursing Minimum Data Set	All Nursing	Clinical Data Elements
NMMDS Nursing Management Minimum Data Set	All Settings	Nursing Administrative Data Elements
Nursing-Developed Terminologies*		
CCC Clinical Care Classification	All Nursing Care	Diagnoses, Interventions, and Outcomes
ICNP® International Classification of Nursing Practice	All Nursing	Diagnoses, Interventions, and Outcomes
NANDA NANDA International	All Nursing	Diagnoses
NIC Nursing Interventions Classification	All Nursing	Interventions
NOC Nursing Outcomes Classification	All Nursing	Outcomes
Omaha System Omaha System	Home Care, Public Health, and Community	Diagnoses, Interventions, and Outcomes
PCDS Patient Care Data Set* (retired)	Acute Care	Diagnoses, Interventions, and Outcomes
10. PNDS Perioperative Nursing Data Set	Perioperative	Diagnoses, Interventions and Outcomes
Multidisciplinary Terminologies		
ABC ABC Codes	Nursing and Other	Interventions
LOINC® Logical Observation Identifiers, Names, and Codes	Nursing and Other	Outcomes and Assessments
SNOMED CT Systematic Nomenclature of Medicine Clinical Terms	Nursing and Other	Diagnoses, Interventions, and Outcomes

Source: ANA 2006a. (* Except for the retired PCDS, all nursing-developed terminologies are still currently in use.)

The content in this appendix is not current and is of historical significance only.

To promote the integration of standardized terminologies into information technology solutions, ANA's Nursing Information and Data Set Evaluation Center (NIDSEC) develops and disseminates standards pertaining to information systems that support the documentation of nursing practice, and evaluates voluntarily submitted information systems against these standards.

At a higher level of structure, several resources facilitate interoperability between different systems of concepts and nomenclature. For instance, the Systematized Nomenclature of Medicine, or SNOMED CT (IHTSDO, 2007), is considered a universal healthcare reference terminology and messaging structure. SNOMED CT enables one nursing terminology system to be mapped to another, e.g., Omaha System with North American Nursing Diagnosis Association (NANDA), Nursing Interventions Classification (NIC), and Nursing Outcomes Classification (NOC). On a larger scale, the Unified Medical Language System (UMLS) of the National Library of Medicine (NLM, 2006) incorporates the work of over one hundred vocabularies, including SNOMED CT. The informatics nurse and informatics nurse specialist must be aware of these tools, and may be called upon to understand the concepts of one or more languages, the relationships between concepts, and integration into existing vocabularies for a given organization.

The importance of languages and vocabularies cannot be overstated. Informatics nurses must seek a broader picture of the implications of their work, and the uses and outcomes of languages and vocabularies for end users. For instance, nurses mapping a home care vocabulary to an intervention vocabulary must see beyond the technical aspect of the work. They must understand that a case manager for a multi-system health organization or a home care agency may be basing knowledge of nursing acuity and case mix on the differing vocabularies that they have integrated. The INS must attempt to envision the varied uses of the data, information, and knowledge that have been created.

Concepts and Tools from Information Science and Computer Science

Tools and methods from computer and information sciences are fundamental to NI, including:

- Information technology
- Information structures

- Information management

- Information communication

Information technology includes computer hardware, software, communication, and network technologies, derived primarily from computer science. The other three elements are derived primarily from information science. Information structures organize data, information, and knowledge for processing by computers. Information management is an elemental process by which one files, stores, and manipulates data for various uses. Information communication enables systems to send data and to present information in a format that improves understanding. The use of information technology distinguishes informatics from more traditional methods of information management.

Human–Computer Interaction and Related Concepts

Human–computer interaction (HCI), usability, and ergonomics are concepts of fundamental interest to the INS. Essentially, HCI deals with people, software applications, computer technology, and the ways they influence each other (Dix, Finlay, Abowd, & Beale, 2004). Elements of HCI are rooted in psychology, social psychology, and cognitive science. However, the design, development, implementation, and evaluation of applications derive from applied work in computer science, a specific discipline (In this case nursing), and information science. For example, an INS would assess a medication ordering application before purchase to determine whether the design complements the way nurses cognitively process orders.

A related concept is usability, which deals with human performance during computer interactions for specific tasks in a specific context. Usability means the efficiency and effectiveness of an application. An INS might study the ease of learning an application, the ease of using it, the speed of task completion, or errors that occur during use when determining which system or application would best fit a nursing unit.

In the United States, the term ergonomics typically is used to describe the design and implementation of equipment, tools, and machines related to human safety, comfort, and convenience. Commonly, the term ergonomics refers to attributes of physical equipment or to principles of arrangement of equipment in the work environment. For instance, an INS may have a role in ensuring that sound ergonomics principles are used in an intensive care unit to select and arrange various devices to support workflow for cross-disciplinary providers as well as patients' families.

HCI, usability, and ergonomics are typically subsumed under the rubric of human factors, or how humans and technology relate to each other. The overall goal is to design software, devices, and equipment to promote optimal task completion. Optimal task completion includes the concepts of efficiency and effectiveness; it also considers the safety of the user. The INS and IN must understand all these concepts to successfully develop, select, implement, and evaluate information structures and informatics solutions.

The importance of human factors in healthcare was elevated with the Institute of Medicine's 2001 report. Before this, HCI and usability assessments and methods were being incorporated into health at a glacial speed. In the past five years the number of HCI and usability publications in healthcare has increased substantially. Vendors have installed usability laboratories and incorporated usability testing of their products into their systems life cycles. The FDA has mandated usability testing as part of their approval process for new devices (FDA, 2007a). Thus, HCI and usability are critical concepts for INs and INSs to understand. Numerous usability methods and tools are available, e.g., heuristics (rules of thumb), naturalistic observation, and think-aloud protocols.

Phenomena of Nursing

The metaparadigm of nursing comprises four key concepts: nurse, person, health, and environment. Nurses make decisions about interventions from their unique perspectives. Nursing actions are based upon the inter-relationships between the concepts and are related to the values nurses hold relative to them. Decision-making is the process of choosing among alternatives. The decisions that nurses make can be characterized by both the quality of decisions and the impact of the actions resulting from those decisions. As knowledge workers, nurses make numerous decisions that affect the life and well-being of individuals, families, and communities. The process of decision-making in nursing is guided by the concept of critical thinking. "Critical thinking is the intellectually disciplined process of actively and skillfully using knowledge to conceptualize, apply, analyze, synthesize, and/or evaluate data and information as a guide to belief and action." (Scriven & Paul, 2003)

The content in this appendix is not current and is of historical significance only.

Clinical wisdom is the ability of the nurse to add experience and intuition to a situation involving the care of a person (Benner, Hooper-Kyriakidis, & Stannard, 1999). Wisdom in informatics is the ability of the informatics nurse specialist to evaluate the documentation drawn from a health information system (HIS) and the ability to adapt or change the system settings or parameters to improve the workflow of the clinical nurse.

Nurses' decision-making can be described as an array of choices that include specific behaviors, as well as cognitive processing of one or more issues. For example, nurses use data transformed into information to determine interventions for persons, families, and communities. Nurses make decisions about potential problems presented by an individual and about recommendations to address those problems. They also make decisions in collaboration with other healthcare professionals such as physicians, pharmacists, or social workers. Decisions also may occur outside the practice environment, as in executive offices, classrooms, and research laboratories.

An information system collects and processes data and information. Decision support systems are computer applications designed to facilitate human decision-making. Decision support systems are typically rule-based: they use a knowledge base and a set of rules to analyze data and information and provide recommendations. Other decision support systems are based on knowledge models induced directly from data, regression, or classification models that predict characteristics or outcomes.

An expert system is a decision support system that implements the knowledge of human experts. Recommendations take the form of alerts, such as calling user attention to abnormal lab results or potential adverse drug events, or suggestions, e.g., appropriate medications, therapies, or other actions (Haug, Gardner, & Evans, 1999). Whereas control systems implement decisions without involvement of a user, decision support systems merely provide recommendations and rely on the wisdom of the user to apply them. As Blum (1986) demonstrated, the concepts of data, information, knowledge, and wisdom exemplify different levels of automated systems. The relationships between these concepts and information, decision support, and expert systems are represented in Figure 3.

The content in this appendix is not current and is of historical significance only.

Figure 3. Levels and Types of Automated Systems

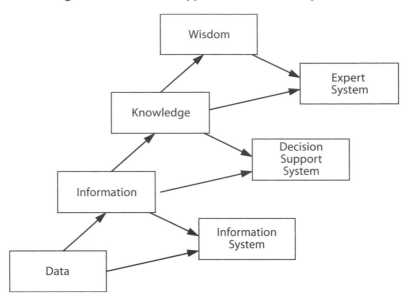

Reprinted from Englebardt & Nelson, 2002, Figure 1-5, page 14 with permission from Elsevier.

In summary, the INS must navigate the complex relationships between the following elements and understand how they facilitate decision-making:

- Data, information, knowledge, and wisdom

- Nursing science, information science, computer science, cognitive science and other sciences of interest

- Nurse, person, health, and environment

- Information structures, information technology, management and communication of information

References: Introduction, Metastructures, Concepts, and Tools

American Nurses Association (ANA). (2006a). *ANA Recognized Terminologies and Data Element Sets*. Retrieved October 10, 2007 from http://nursingworld.org/npii/terminologies.htm

The content in this appendix is not current and is of historical significance only.

Benner, P.E., Hooper-Kyriakidis, P.L., & Stannard, D. (1999). *Clinical wisdom and interventions in critical care: A thinking-in-action approach.* Philadelphia: W.B. Saunders.

Bellinger, G., Castro, D., & Mills, A. (2004). Data, information, knowledge, and wisdom. Retrieved October 10, 2007 from http://www.systems-thinking.org/dikw/dikw.htm

Blum, B. (1986). *Clinical information systems.* New York: Springer-Verlag.

Clark, D. (2004) The continuum of understanding. From *The way of systems.* Retrieved October 10, 2007 from http://www.nwlink.com/~donclark/performance/understanding.html.

Dix, A., Finlay, J., Abowd, G., & Beale, R. (2004). *Human-computer interaction.* Harlow, England: Pearson, Prentice Hall.

Englebardt, S. & Nelson, R. (2002) *Health care informatics: An interdisciplinary approach.* St. Louis: Mosby-Year Book, Inc.

Graves, J., & Corcoran, S. (1989). The study of nursing informatics. *Image, 21*(4), 227–230.

Harrison, L. (2002). Nursing activity in general intensive care. *Journal of Clinical Nursing, 11*(2), 158–67.

Haug, P., Gardner, R., & Evans, S. (1999). Hospital-based decision support. In E.S. Berner (Ed.), Clinical *Decision Support Systems: Theory and Practice*, pp. 77–104. New York: Springer-Verlag.

Hendrickson, G. (1990). How do nurses use their time? *Journal of Nursing Administration, 20*(3), 31–38.

Institute of Medicine (IOM). (2001). *Crossing the quality chasm: A new health system for the 21st century.* Washington, DC: National Academies Press.

International Health Terminology Standards Development Organization (IHTSDO). (2007). *SNOMED-CT.* Retrieved October 10, 2007 from http://www.ihtsdo.org/.

The content in this appendix is not current and is of historical significance only.

Jinks, A.M. (2000) What do nurses do? An observational survey of the activities of nurses on acute surgical and rehabilitative wards. *Journal of Nursing Management 8*(5), 273–279.

Jydstrup, R.A., & J.J.Gross. (1966) Cost of information handling in hospitals. *Health Services Research 1*(3): 235–271.

Nelson, R., & Joos, I. (1989). On language in nursing: From data to wisdom. *PLN Vision.* p. 6.

Norrie, P. (1997). Nurses' time management in intensive care. *Nursing Critical Care*, 2(3), 121–125.

Norrie, P. (1999) The parameters that cardiothoracic intensive care nurses use to assess the progress or deterioration of their patients. *Nursing Critical Care*, 4(3), 133–137.

Scriven, M., & Paul, R. (2003). Defining critical thinking. Santa Rosa, CA.: Foundation for Critical Thinking. Retrieved December 13, 2007 from http://www.criticalthinking.org

Staggers, N., & Thompson, C.B. (2002). The evolution of definitions for nursing informatics: A critical analysis and revised definition. *Journal of the American Medical Informatics Association*, 33(1), 75–81.

Turley, J.P. (1996). Toward a model for nursing informatics. *Image: Journal of Nursing Scholarship*, 28(4), 309–313.

Zielstorff, R.D. (1981). How computer systems influence nursing activities in hospitals. In *The Proceedings of the First National Conference: Computer Technology and Nursing*, pp. 1–6. Bethesda, MD: National Institutes of Health.

The content in this appendix is not current and is of historical significance only.

Functional Areas for Nursing Informatics

Two recent studies illuminate the current work of INs. Newbold (personal communication, January 17, 2006) created a database of job titles for nurses working in informatics beginning in the early 1980s. As of early 2006, the database included titles for 6338 members of nursing and informatics organizations, conference attendees and participants on NI electronic discussion lists. However, the top 50 job titles did not consistently map to their responsibilities and activities. INs with different titles may actually be performing the same functions, and INs with the same titles may perform very different functions.

A 2007 Health Information Management and Systems Society (HIMSS) survey of 776 informatics nurses categorized NI work into job responsibilities as opposed to job titles (HIMSS, 2007). The top job responsibility of respondents was systems implementation (45%), down from 67% in 2004. The second and third top job responsibilities reported by HIMSS respondents were system development (41%) and liaison (35%).

Not only are there assorted titles and activities within nursing informatics, the environments in which INSs and INs practice are many and evolving. Initially, NI focused nearly exclusively on the hospital setting. Now INs work in such diverse settings as home health and hospice agencies, nursing homes, public and community health agencies, physician offices, and ambulatory care centers. They are employed by medical device vendors, large and small software companies, web content providers, disease management companies, and government agencies, in numerous settings (Sensmeier, West, & Horowicz, 2004). Across environments , INSs and INs commonly practice in interdisciplinary healthcare environments and are often expected to interact with information technology (IT) professionals during all phases of the systems life cycle. And more commonly than in the past, INs may be the IT professionals themselves.

Nursing informatics supports multiple constituencies and stakeholders such as cross-disciplinary team members, healthcare consumers, information technology professionals, and healthcare agencies and organizations. INSs are particularly well suited to work in multidisciplinary and interdisciplinary environments. After all, nurses have planned, implemented, and coordinated activities involving multiple constituencies in a consumer-centered fashion from their earliest days.

INSs use scientific and informatics principles. More importantly, they employ creative strategies in meaningful informatics solutions. INSs also bring unique perspectives of cross-disciplinary work, solid understanding of operational processes, and the value of consumer advocacy to informatics functions. INs and INSs may find that they need varying kinds of advanced preparation to match the informatics project at hand. For instance, an INS coordinating the implementation of a learning management system may benefit from advanced preparation in adult education.

Many registered nurses have worked on informatics initiatives for many years and have built their knowledge base and expertise from on-the-job experience. The evolving mandate for electronic information systems and the increasing complexity of healthcare services and practice have raised the bar for the nursing professional. Select informatics competencies will soon be required in all undergraduate and graduate nursing curricula. Accredited graduate level educational programs for this specialty nursing practice were first offered in 1989 and are now more widely available, especially through distance education and online programs. Rather than offer discipline-specific informatics programs, some universities have elected to embrace an interdisciplinary approach and offer graduate studies in health informatics or bioinformatics. A graduate level informatics degree is becoming the standard.

Professional certification as an informatics nurse became a reality in late 1995 when the American Nurses Credentialing Center (ANCC) offered the nursing informatics certification exam as its first computer-based examination. Informatics nurses and informatics nurse specialists may elect to pursue other pertinent certifications in areas such as project management, security and privacy, network management, and knowledge management. Employers are beginning to use certification as a preferred characteristic during the hiring process.

Because of the tendency to confuse roles with titles and the vast number of position titles and lack of standardization among them, this section describes the *functional areas* for INSs and INs. The following present overall functional areas of nursing informatics:

- Administration, leadership, and management
- Analysis
- Compliance and integrity management

The content in this appendix is not current and is of historical significance only.

- Consultation

- Coordination, facilitation, and integration

- Development

- Educational and professional development

- Policy development and advocacy

- Research and evaluation

The last discussion in this section describes integrated functions, especially those crossing clinical practice and informatics. INSs may be in positions that focus primarily in one functional area, or, more frequently, several functional areas are combined within a particular NI position.

Administration, Leadership, and Management

As is true of administration in general, leadership and management functions in nursing informatics consist of both higher-level and mid-level administrative functions (ANA, 2004b). Increasingly, INSs are attaining senior leadership positions. Positions may be titled President, Director, Chief Information Officer (CIO), or similar leadership titles (AMIA, 2006a; Staggers & Lasome, 2005; Greene, 2004). In this functional capacity, nursing informatics leaders are expected to be visionary and establish the direction of large-scale informatics solutions. The nursing informatics leader often serves as a catalyst for developing strategic plans, creating national or system policies and procedures, and serving as champion for complex projects and disparate system users.

In mid-level management, INSs may supervise resources and activities for all phases of the systems life cycle. These activities may include needs analysis, requirements gathering, design, development, selection and purchase, testing, implementation, and evaluation of systems to support all facets of nursing and healthcare delivery. In all levels, leadership combines the skills of superb communication, change management, risk assessment, and coalition building with political finesse, business acumen, and strategic application knowledge.

INSs serving in this functional area may put most of their energy into leadership and management. In other positions, administration may be part of a position merged with other functional areas. Examples might include:

- INS at a large hospital system, supervising an implementation and education team, representing nursing interests on various IT committees, performing project management for multiple documentation projects, and having oversight of nursing standards and vocabularies used in applications.

- Project director for a clinical software company, managing implementation teams for various client projects (hospitals to ambulatory facilities) and consulting with clients on all aspects of systems selection, customization, adoption, and use of software.

- Grants administrator for an information science research agency seeking and writing grants that would fund NI-related projects, designing budgets, and ensuring optimal allocation of resources.

Analysis

Data can be aggregated and analyzed in an infinite number of ways to synthesize knowledge, inform decision support and outcomes management, and advance the science of nursing informatics. The INS may use a number of tools to accomplish these ends. Taxonomies and clinical vocabularies can be used to tag consumer data for higher-level analysis. Meta-analysis can identify large-scale trends across multiple groups of data. Systems and requirements analysis can track the flow of data in a system, customized to end-user needs. Workflow analysis can detail steps taken for a number of tasks.

A major responsibility of the INS is to understand work process flows, the particular informatics solution, and how these affect each other. Processes must be designed for successful interactions between users and computers. Competency in formal systems analysis techniques and use of statistical software may be required. These techniques compare the capabilities and limitations of systems to be installed, and where changes must be designed. Discrepancies between the current and ideal systems must be identified and redundancies removed. The clinical analysis process also may include tools and systematic methods, such as process redesign, to enhance safety and reduce inefficiencies.

INSs may also engage in the process of knowledge discovery in databases (KDD). Using sound methodologies and practical evidence-based recommendations, the INS can discover information and knowledge related to diverse areas of nursing practice. Knowledge discovery

The content in this appendix is not current and is of historical significance only.

methods, including data mining and machine learning methods, can be applied along with statistical analysis and data visualization techniques, to identify and understand patterns in very large data stores, such as enterprise data warehouses (Fayyad, 1996).

Analysis is also required with languages and taxonomies. Nursing languages such as Nursing Interventions Classification (NIC), Nursing Outcomes Classification (NOC), and medical vocabularies must be periodically re-evaluated for their applicability and currency (CNCCE, 2004). Analysis of a meta-database such as the Unified Medical Language System or UMLS (NLM, 2006) requires knowledge of nursing as well as medical vocabularies in order to analyze groups of taxonomies, a task ideally suited to the expertise of an INS.

Analysis of outcomes may be related to any domain of nursing practice—clinical, education, research, or administration. The complexity and levels of outcomes must be determined for healthcare consumers, populations, and institutions. Analysis can include the use of Human-Computer Interaction (HCI) principles and methods. In that domain, INSs use HCI tools and methods such as heuristics and cognitive walk-through to analyze the fit of users, tasks, and contexts. Other tools are also available. Analysts use system tools to maintain data integrity and reliability, facilitate data aggregation and analysis, identify outcomes, and develop performance measurements. These techniques allow nurses to contribute to building a knowledge base consisting of the data, information, theories, and models used by nurses and other stakeholders in decision-making and support of healthcare. Analysis activities may include:

- A nursing analyst in a hospice setting tracks health consumer data to establish a weighted case mix to determine nursing personnel allocations.

- A quality improvement (QI) specialist in a hospital system aggregates multi-site research data related to diagnosis and nursing procedures.

- A quality assurance (QA) analyst works with nurse managers to re-tool current work processes after examining existing system data in customized QA reports.

- An analyst applies knowledge discovery methods to warehoused electronic data to build a predictive model of patient falls.

The content in this appendix is not current and is of historical significance only.

Compliance and Integrity Management

With the advent of national laws advocating for the protection of health information, INSs are responsible for ensuring the ethical use of data, as well as data integrity, security, and confidentiality of protected health information. One function of the INS is knowledge and application of ethical standards. The Health Insurance Portability and Accountability Act (HIPAA) of 1996 has obliged healthcare organizations to revise operational procedures for staff, as well as technical processes, to maintain compliance. INSs must be fluent in these new requirements; they are involved in creating, implementing, and assuring organizational change to meet new legislative mandates. Compliance also includes adherence to national and international standards. These standards may include those from government agencies, such as the Food and Drug Administration (FDA) and National Institutes of Health (NIH), as well as accreditation organizations such as the Joint Commission.

Ethical issues related to consumer privacy abound. One arises from knowledge discovery in databases (KDD), where prediction of outcomes based on individual characteristics, behavior, or usage may be used to stratify groups of people. Although used in a variety of industries, KDD remains controversial in health care. Adequate HIPAA protections must be in place, and relevant ethical issues must be considered in all phases of data retrieval and analysis. For example, analysis of genomic data may result in sensitive predictions of susceptibility to disease. Given the explosive growth of large data stores and enterprise data warehouses, KDD is important for extraction of useful information and knowledge; nevertheless, protecting consumer privacy is vital. The INS can help ensure a balance between access and privacy.

The emerging sciences of genomics and bioinformatics could be used to predict risk for certain diseases, and thus insurability risk. Ethical issues surround the use of new products, such as embedded technologies and radio-frequency identification (RFID) and their application in caring for persons with Alzheimer's disease and other dementias. As the profession matures, some of these issues will be resolved and standards will be established. Requirements will continue to evolve; see the section, Future of NI, on page 61. Examples of compliance and integrity management activities include:

- The security officer for a hospital ensures that HIPAA standards are met by software vendors within the organization, periodically

The content in this appendix is not current and is of historical significance only.

monitors software audit logs for breaches, and ensures that passwords are not shared and backup and disaster procedures are in place and operational.

- A compliance officer for a state health agency writes and enforces policies that conform to state and national laws respecting records retention.

- A care coordinator administrator for a hospital system ensures the confidentiality of data transmitted via telehealth and telemedicine devices

Consultation

Informatics nurses and informatics nurse specialists apply informatics knowledge and skills to serve as a resource to clients, both formally and informally, in external and internal settings. Consultants are experts in the areas of process redesign, strategic IT planning, system implementation, writing informatics publications, evaluating clinical software products, working with clients to write requests for proposals, performing market research, and assisting in the planning of conferences, academic courses, and professional development programs. These expert INSs may work for a consulting firm, be employed as staff of the organization where they consult, own an independent practice, or be recognized as an expert by writing about NI and speaking at NI-related events. Flexibility, good communication skills, breadth and depth of clinical and informatics knowledge, and excellent interpersonal skills are needed to respond to rapidly changing projects and demands. Examples include:

- Consulting with individuals and groups in defining healthcare information problems and identifying methods for implementing, utilizing, and modifying IT solutions and data structures to support healthcare access, delivery, and evaluation.

- Consulting as the project manager, ensuring that team members are performing duties as assigned and the project is completed within budget.

- Consulting with clients in writing requests for proposals to elicit vendor bids for informatics solutions and in evaluating vendor responses.

Coordination, Facilitation, and Integration

One of the most common NI roles is implementing informatics solutions. Nurses are particularly well suited for IT implementation, as it essentially follows the nursing process of assessment, planning, implementation, and evaluation (ANA, 2004a). Also, the INS frequently serves as a bridge between informatics solution users and IT experts. The IN or INS serves as project coordinator, facilitating change management and integrating the information and technology to transform processes. In this role, project management knowledge and skills are essential to the successful outcome of the project. Project coordination can range from small, department-centered applications to enterprise-wide electronic health record (EHR) installations, from coordinating a rehabilitation module in the rehabilitation unit to installing a complete EHR in 42 hospitals.

Of particular note, effective communication is an inherent part of many NI functions, but especially related to coordination, facilitation, and integration. The IN and INS are at the hub of cross-disciplinary communication among professional disciplines and IT, serving as translators and integrators for system requirements and impacts.

In another instance, informatics nurses serve as the liaison between software engineers and end users. In this capacity, the informatics nurse ensures that the necessary testing or research is performed to determine the end user's needs, and that this information is conveyed to the software engineers in terms they can understand. Once the engineer has created a product, the INS evaluates the utility of the product from the viewpoint of the end user. This liaison type of facilitation and coordination occurs in multiple environments. Ensuring the integration of nursing vocabularies and standardized nomenclatures in applications is another example. In this case INSs also act as usability experts and recommend ideal formats for the utilization of technology. Examples of coordination, facilitation, and integration might include:

- The project coordinator for a statewide electronic medical record implementation coordinates all aspects of the project and supervises a cross-disciplinary team to train public health personnel to use the application.

- The project manager for a clinical software company manages the resources and activities using tools such as project management software and project plans for clients whose responsibilities cross inpatient and ambulatory areas

- The clinical liaison for a telehealth software vendor communicates with providers and consumers to ensure that all parties are agreeable to development and implementation plans, and ensures that providers using the system receive adequate technical education.

- A usability expert on a software development team advises software engineers on screen design from the standpoint of clinical documentation needs, performs or coordinates testing of iterative designs, and validates clinical requirements with the users.

Development

Development was listed as the second most common responsibility of HIMSS NI respondents in 2007 (HIMSS, 2007). A developer is responsible for translating user requirements into effective informatics solutions. INSs are involved in a vast array of development activities, from conceptualizing models for applications, to software and hardware design, to the design of education manuals, to the design of complex technology networks. As part of this function, INSs and INs participate in the process of design, iterative development, testing, and dissemination of quality informatics solutions for nurses, interdisciplinary providers, and consumers. An understanding of the information needs of nurses and the nursing profession, consumers and consumer care processes, as well as knowledge of business, client services, projected market directions, product design, product development methods, market research, contemporary programming, systems design, and modeling language are essential for practicing in a development environment.

Adherence to national standards and regulatory requirements is also essential to any development work. In order to ensure interoperability between systems, INSs and INs involved in system development must be knowledgeable about international standards requirements. Existing standards include Health Level Seven (HL-7), International Organization for Standardization (ISO), Current Procedural Terminology (CPT), International Classification of Disease (ICD), and Digital Image Communication (DICOM) group standards, as well as Section 508 accessibility standards (Hammond, 1995; GSA, 2006). An understanding of the current work on standards is mandatory. Development responsibilities might include:

- A developer with a personal health record software vendor creates user-friendly screens for consumers to enter information as well as screens for nurses to display and interpret the data.

- A database administrator with a large multi-site teaching organization manages an expanded nursing vocabulary set for inpatient, ambulatory, and home health nursing documentation.

- A nurse web content developer for a consortium creates and validates content for educational handouts, help and tool tips for user interfaces that display national guidelines, and educational tools. This would include new and innovative tools for knowledge dissemination.

- A programmer in a hospital IT department codes software for documenting diabetic education.

Education and Professional Development

Education is a critical component of many NI functions and may directly affect the success or failure of any new or modified IT solution. Vendors of information systems frequently use the term *training* when referring to client education. In nursing, however, the broader label of *education* is used. Adherence to solid educational principles is a component of education and professional development (ANA, 2000). Teaching nurses and nursing students, healthcare consumers, and other interdisciplinary health team members about the effective and ethical uses of information technology, as well as NI concepts and theories, is essential for the optimal use of informatics solutions in nursing practice. Ever-changing requirements in health information technology make continuing education essential as well. INSs and INs in this capacity develop, implement, and evaluate educational curricula and educational technologies that meet the needs of students.

In this role, educators and trainers assess and evaluate informatics skills and competencies while providing feedback to students regarding the effectiveness of the learning activity and the students' ability to demonstrate newly acquired skills. Educators and trainers manage, evaluate, report, and utilize data and information related to students and the educational delivery system. These INSs are innovators in defining and developing educational technologies, integrating the solutions into the educational and practice environments, and challenging organizations to consider and adopt innovative informatics solutions.

The content in this appendix is not current and is of historical significance only.

The INS must consider information competency as well as literacy. Computer literacy is a core competency needed in health care, and should be taught in nursing curricula at all levels. In addition, information literacy must be integrated into practice and used to support knowledge management. These are the foundations of informatics competencies.

Education and professional development includes not only INSs, INs, and end users, but also consumers. With the advent of distance technologies such as telehealth and Internet-based consumer-accessible applications, new competencies are needed to ensure that health information is displayed to consumers at an appropriate level of understanding; support staff may not be available in person. Cultural issues, language considerations, and literacy of consumers may not be apparent, and materials may need to be more fully assessed for appropriate presentation and understanding.

INSs may need to ensure presentation of content for web-based knowledge portals of private and government health organizations that may exist in multiple locations, or only virtually. Health information may need to be distilled for consumer consumption. Thus education and professional development involve not only educating INs and INSs, but also developing appropriate interfaces for the consumer. Education and professional development might include:

- A professor of nursing at a major university teaches graduate nursing students enrolled in a nursing informatics degree program or teaches nursing students at all levels the basic NI principles and foundations.

- A clinical preceptor for newly hired nurses and students provides orientation about telehealth, engages them in using telehealth technology, and role models the telehealth nurse responsibilities of monitoring physiologic parameters and providing consumer education.

- An educator for a vendor travels internationally to train nurses on the product's operations, capabilities, troubleshooting, limitations, and benefits.

- A staff development liaison for a large hospital educates nurses and other end users about how to integrate clinical applications into their work processes.

- A help desk team member for a large oncology center works with users as product upgrades are released, answers clinical user questions on the phone or in person, and trouble-shoots user problems.

- A patient education coordinator facilitates electronic consumer health resources.

- A web developer is responsible for development, maintenance, and presentation of disease content for a hospital web portal.

Policy Development and Advocacy

INSs play a key role in formulation of health policy, particularly bringing expertise in data and information content, data structures, and IT solutions with those attributes. Policy development may be at any level—international, national, state, professional specialty, institution or a work unit. INSs are experts in defining the data needed and the structure, management, and availability of those data for decision-making. As such, they advocate for consumers, providers, and the enterprise, and articulate relevant issues from a nursing perspective. Policy-related activities may include developing, writing, implementing, and evaluating guidance. Regardless of the level or activity, INSs are partners in setting health policy, particularly related to information management and communication, infrastructure development, and economics.

The advocacy function of the INS or IN also encompasses consumer health. INs may be part of initiatives such as promoting the adoption of technology for rural programs to increase access to health services. Advocacy may include educating legislators about increasing telecommunication access, expanding reimbursement for technology-enabled consumer services, or educating the public on ways to access health-related materials via the Internet. Examples of policy development and advocacy function of the INS or IN might include:

- The president of a health information management organization represents nursing on a national information standards task force.

- A lobbyist participates in advocacy efforts on behalf of consumers for increased government funding of demonstration or pilot informatics projects.

- A president of a nursing informatics organization writes letters to elected officials to obtain their support for reimbursement of services by remote, technology-enabled providers.

The content in this appendix is not current and is of historical significance only.

Research and Evaluation

INSs conduct research into the design, development, and implementation of informatics solutions, and their impact on users, such as healthcare organizations, providers, consumers, and payers. INS researchers use systematic methods of inquiry (including traditional and newer techniques) to identify and evaluate data, information, knowledge, and wisdom in informatics solutions and data repositories. Research and evaluation functions include, but are not limited to:

- Research in concept or symbolic representation of nursing phenomena
- Evaluation of clinical decision-making in nursing
- Applied research in development, implementation, usability, and outcome implications of solutions
- Consumers' and interdisciplinary providers' use of health information tools and resources
- Evaluation of effective methods for information systems implementation, acceptance, and utilization
- Human factors or ergonomics research into the design of systems and their impact on interdisciplinary providers, consumers, nurses, and their interactions
- Evaluation research on the effects of systems on the processes and outcomes of consumer care
- Usability testing of nursing and consumer applications
- Evaluating how consumers utilize computerized healthcare products
- Research in clinical vocabularies
- Interaction of consumers, providers, and technology
- Consumer communication and usage of technology-based support groups

Research in nursing informatics can span a range of activities, from experimental research to process improvement and informal evaluation to evidence-based practice. Much of the work is innovative and may be initiated by INSs or conducted at the request of an organization or agency. INSs working in research and evaluation might conduct research projects to develop and refine standardized nursing vocabularies, or link nursing interventions to outcomes in large data sets. This work is essential in defining, describing, and evaluating data, information, knowledge, and wisdom. It may include the evaluation of organizational attributes for successful adoption of documentation systems or the impact and efficacy of hardware and software solutions.

Nursing informatics research may also incorporate a consumer orientation. It may study effective nurse-consumer interactions in web-based interactions with older consumers, or the impact of new applications on nurses' workflow. Patient reactions to instant messaging from providers may be studied. Examples of the research function of the INS include:

- The chief for nursing research for a large software company oversees projects to evaluate the impact of enterprise electronic health records on patient care outcomes.

- A nursing informatics analyst in a hospital IT department aggregates data about the incidence of decubiti, creates trend reports and predictive models for nurse managers, and analyzes outcomes against quality indicators.

- A nurse researcher conducts a usability study comparing consumer entry of information at a clinic-based kiosk to in-person interviews.

Integrated Functional Areas: Telehealth and Telenursing as Exemplar

Informatics solutions are foundational support for healthcare delivery. In some cases, however, informatics solutions are more tightly integrated with care delivery. Clinical care and informatics intersect in areas such as telehealth and radiation oncology and serve as examples of integrated functional areas. In the discussion below, telehealth serves as the exemplar.

Telehealth, as defined by the U.S. Office for the Advancement of Telehealth, is "the use of electronic information and telecommunications technologies to support long-distance clinical healthcare, patient and professional health-related education, public health and health administration" (HRSA, 2001). Telenursing is the use of distance or telecommunications technologies by nurses to monitor consumer and public health and administrative functions, as well as deliver healthcare education (Milholland, 2000; NCSNB, 2003). With the widespread expansion of telehealth technologies, standards have been developed that take into account differing countries' cultures and governance standards

The content in this appendix is not current and is of historical significance only.

(Milholland-Hunter, 2001). Standards may pertain to the transmission of data and information as well as protocols for providing care.

Nursing informatics primarily fulfills a clinical support role, as opposed to a direct clinical practice role. Telehealth is primarily a clinical practice role, with technical aspects required to deliver care. The 2004 International Telenursing Survey (Grady, Schlachta-Fairchild, & Elfrink, 2005) surveyed international telenurses worldwide. Of the 719 participants, only 18 had informatics in their job titles. Within this group, over half were advanced practice clinicians. Ten of the clinicians had the term informatics in their titles. Thus, the interface between nursing informatics and telehealth nursing today primarily occurs at the technical or support level. In the future, telehealth may evolve toward an emphasis on information (versus technology), and informatics principles, methods, and tools may expand in the future.

Standards for telehealth nursing clinical practice are outlined in *ANA's Core Principles on Telehealth* (1998) and *Competencies for Telehealth Technologies in Nursing* (1999). These describe the interface between telehealth and informatics, referring to the technical aspects of telehealth as clinical support and telehealth as clinical practice. Examples of the telehealth role of the IN or INS might be:

- A telehealth network coordinator for a rural telehealth program ensures the appropriate deployment of technology, and customization for distance-related needs.

- A program manager for telehealth in a home health agency organizes the integration of telehealth into the agency's operations, supports the alignment of telehealth technology with the overall technology strategy of the agency, leads the adoption and implementation of the program, and evaluates and maintains telehealth outcomes and accountability for those outcomes (Starren et al., 2005).

- A nurse researcher conducting a program evaluation compares the impact of an online, telehealth cardiac education program to that of an in-person support group on level of depression and adherence to diet.

NI Functional Areas: Conclusions

With the continued miniaturization of technology, as well as developments in information science and nursing science, NI functions will

The content in this appendix is not current and is of historical significance only.

continue to expand, evolving into functions not yet envisioned. INSs and INs will need to continually assess new knowledge management and technology trends and incorporate them into their own practices. Integrated functional areas will continue to expand. The functional areas listed here will be combined with new areas to create innovative positions of the future.

References: Functional Areas

American Medical Informatics Association (AMIA). (2006a). Nursing Informatics Working Group. *Roles in nursing informatics*. Retrieved October 10, 2007 from http://www.amia.org/mbrcenter/wg/ni/roles/inf_nrs.asp

American Nurses Association (ANA). (1998). *Core principles on telehealth*. Washington, DC: American Nurses Publishing.

American Nurses Association (ANA). (1999). *Competencies for telehealth technologies in nursing*. Washington, DC: American Nurses Publishing.

American Nurses Association (ANA). (2000). *Scope and standards of practice for nursing professional development*. Washington, DC: American Nurses Publishing.

American Nurses Association (ANA). (2004a). *Nursing scope and standards of practice*. Silver Spring, MD: Nursesbooks.org.

American Nurses Association (ANA). (2004b). *Scope and standards for nurse administrators* (2nd ed.). Silver Spring, MD: Nursesbooks.org.

Bellinger, G., Castro, D., & Mills, A. (2004). Data, information, knowledge, and wisdom. Retrieved October 10, 2007 from http://www.systems-thinking.org/dikw/dikw.htm

Center for Nursing Classification and Clinical Effectiveness (CNCCE). (2004). *Overview of NIC/NOC*. Retrieved October 10, 2007 from http://www.nursing.uiowa.edu/excellence/nursing_knowledge/clinical_effectiveness/index.htm

The content in this appendix is not current and is of historical significance only.

General Services Administration (GSA). (2006). Office of Government-wide Policy, IT Accessibility & Workforce Division (ITAW). *Section 508.* Retrieved October 10, 2007 from http://www.section508.gov.

Fayyad, U. (1996). Data mining and knowledge discovery: Making sense out of data. *IEEE Expert 11*(5), 220–225. Retrieved December 13, 2007, from http://www.aaai.org/AITopics/assets/PDF/AIMag17-03-2-article.pdf.

Grady, J., Schlachta-Fairchild, L. & Elfrink, V. (2005). Results of the 2004 International Telenursing Survey. *Telemedicine and e-Health, 11*(2), 197.

Greene, J. (2004). RN to CIO: High-tech nurses bridge hospitals' cultural divide. *Hospitals and Health Networks 78*(2):40–46.

Hammond, W.E. (1995). *Glossary for healthcare standards.* Retrieved February 28, 2006 from http://dmi-www.mc.duke.edu/dukemi/acronyms.htm.

Health Insurance Portability and Accountability Act of 1996 (HIPAA). Retrieved October 10, 2007 from http://aspe.hhs.gov/admnsimp/pl104191.htm.

Health Resources and Services Administration (HRSA). (2001). Office for the Advancement of Telehealth. *Report to Congress on telemedicine.* Retrieved October 10, 2007 from http://www.hrsa.gov/telehealth/pubs/report2001.htm.

Healthcare Information and Management Systems Society (HIMSS). (2007). *2007 HIMSS nursing informatics survey.* Retrieved October 10, 2007 from http://www.himss.org/content/files/surveyresults/2007NursingInformatics.pdf.

Milholland, K. (2000). *Telenursing, telehealth. Nursing and technology advance together.* Geneva: International Council of Nurses.

Milholland-Hunter, K. (2001). *International professional standards for telenursing programmes.* Geneva: International Council of Nurses.

The content in this appendix is not current and is of historical significance only.

National Council of State Boards of Nursing (NCSBN). (2003). *Position paper on telenursing: A challenge to regulation.* Retrieved October 10, 2007 from http://www.ncsbn.org/pdfs/TelenursingPaper.pdf

National Library of Medicine (NLM). (2006). *Unified Medical Language System.* Retrieved October 10, 2007 from http://www.nlm.nih.gov/research/umls.

Newbold, S. K. (2006). Nursing informatics database—Job titles as of January 17, 2006. Electronic correspondence. Email to snewbold@umaryland.edu.

Sensmeier, J., West, L., & Horowicz, J.K. (2004). Survey reveals, role, compensation of nurse informaticists. *Computers, Informatics, Nursing 22*(3), 171, 178–181.

Staggers, N, & Lasome, C. F. (2005). RN, CIO: An executive informatics career. *Computer, Informatics, Nursing 23*(4), 201–206.

Starren, J., Tsai, C., Bakken, S., Aidala, A., Morin, P., Hilliman, C., et al. (2005). The role of nurses installing telehealth technology in the home. *Computers, Informatics, Nursing, 23*(4), 181–189.

Willson, D., Bjornstad, G., Lussier, J., Matney, S., Miller, S., Nelson, N., et al. (2000). Nursing informatics career opportunities. In B. Carty (ed.), *Nursing informatics: education for practice.* New York: Springer.

Informatics Competencies

Because of the increased visibility of information and technology in healthcare settings and complementary educational programs, many stakeholders are faced with a need to define informatics competencies for nurses. Human resource managers and educational planners are just two examples of stakeholders who have an interest in competencies for nursing informatics.

Since 2000, researchers and professional organizations have completed substantial work in defining nursing informatics competencies (Androwich et al., 2003; Curran, 2003; Desjardins et al., 2003; HIMSS, 2005;

The content in this appendix is not current and is of historical significance only.

Jiang, Chen, & Chen, 2004; Staggers, Gassert, & Curran, 2000, 2001, 2002). Several lists of informatics competencies are available, especially those geared toward nurses' educational levels.

Stakeholders such as employers and educators are keenly interested in identifying informatics competencies for various nursing roles. For the discussion here, competencies for typical nursing informatics roles are especially pertinent. To this end, a matrix has been developed, based upon a thorough literature review and the work from a consensus panel. This text and accompanying matrix (Table 2) suggests competencies for typical nursing informatics functional areas discussed in the previous section.

The Intersection of Informatics Competencies and NI Functional Areas

Staggers, Gassert, and Curran (2000, 2001, 2002) studied the relationships between nursing roles and informatics competencies for nurses at four levels of practice: beginning, experienced, INS, and informatics innovator. This framework aligns with educational requirements for all nursing specialties at the beginning and experienced levels, and then identifies specific competencies for the specialty roles of INS and the informatics innovator. Their work not only promoted the integration of informatics competencies into educational curricula, but also influenced policy documents.

To date, the majority of authors have focused on the competencies needed for nursing curricula. Curran (2003) identified informatics competencies for nurse practitioners at Columbia University School of Nursing. Desjardins, Cook, Jenkins, and Bakken (2005) focused on beginning nurse competencies, expanding them to include the knowledge and skills for information literacy to support evidenced-based practice. Like Staggers et al. (2002), this study also linked competencies to four levels of nursing practice. Barton (2005) presented a similar view of informatics competencies for the beginning nurse, identifying a need for competencies in technology or computer literacy as well as information literacy for undergraduate nursing programs.

McNeil, Elfrink, Pierce, Beyea, Bickford, and Averill (2005) examined educational content for required informatics competencies. They asked the deans and directors of 672 baccalaureate and above education programs to describe informatics content taught in their undergraduate and graduate programs. Twenty-five unique content areas were identi-

The content in this appendix is not current and is of historical significance only.

fied for undergraduate (i.e., beginning nurse) and graduate (i.e., experienced nurse) levels of practice. Among the top-ranked competencies for both programs were: a) accessing electronic resources, b) ethical use of information systems, c) evidence-based practice skills, and d) skills for computer-based patient records. The undergraduate program respondents more often identified basic hardware and software skills, whereas the graduate program respondents included competencies related to innovation and change theory, national health database knowledge, and general systems theory.

Jiang, Chen, and Chen (2004) surveyed Taiwanese nursing education programs ranging from non-vocational and vocational nursing programs to collegiate programs for two-, four-, five-year, and graduate-level programs. The authors identified seven domains of competencies and linked them to differing levels of nursing education in Taiwan. In contrast to work in the United States, they identified domains mostly related to computer versus information literacy, including hardware, software, and network concepts; principles of computer application; skills in computer usage; program design; limitations of the computer; personal and social issues; and attitudes toward the computer.

New categories and concomitant competencies for education, as well as practice, are also available. Androwich et al. (2003) described NI competencies needed to improve patient safety and expand nursing practice. Garde, Harrison, and Hovenga (2005) reported specific competencies for:

- Nursing informatics knowledge and skills (e.g., health information systems, electronic patient records, telehealth).

- Information technology knowledge and skills (e.g., programming principles, software development, methodologies and processes, system analysis and design, database design and management).

- Knowledge and skills in organizational and human behavior (e.g., project management, inter-professional communication, risk management, policies and procedures).

- Clinical and health-related knowledge and skills (e.g., evidence based practice, clinical guidelines, care pathways).

The Healthcare Leadership Alliance (HLA) announced the creation of the HLA Competency Directory in the fall of 2005. This directory (HLA,

The content in this appendix is not current and is of historical significance only.

2005) identifies 300 competencies across multiple healthcare management roles, categorized into five domains:

- Leadership
- Communications and relationship management
- Professionalism
- Business knowledge and skills
- Knowledge of the healthcare environment

This directory may be especially pertinent for interdisciplinary settings.

A New Competencies Matrix

The competencies matrix in Table 2 (on page 38 and 39) is derived from Staggers, Gassert, and Curran (2002) and other authors mentioned earlier, and from the ANCC NI Certification exam (ANCC, 2007). These competencies are categorized in three overall areas: Computer Literacy, Information Literacy, and Professional Development/Leadership. Computer literacy competencies relate to the psychomotor use of computers and other technological equipment (Barton, 2005). Information literacy competencies deal with information retrieval knowledge and skills: knowing when there is a need for information; identifying the information needed to address a given problem or issue; finding the needed information and evaluating it; organizing the information; and using the information effectively to address the problem or issue. (ALA, 2006). Professional development and leadership competencies refer to the ethical, procedural, safety, and management issues for informatics solutions in nursing practice, education, research, and administration.

The horizontal axis of the matrix is based on the four educational levels as well as the NI functional areas defined earlier. It is important to recognize that informatics competencies need to be integrated into all educational levels. The panel identified competency foci for each functional area indicated by an **X**. Competencies cross the different nursing informatics functional areas. Although each sub-heading includes more granular competencies beneath it, nurses would not necessarily be expected to achieve every competency within a sub-heading. The areas identified by the **X** merely indicate an area of emphasis.

The absence of an **X** does not mean that the skill is completely irrelevant to that role; rather it means that the skill may not be emphasized in a particular functional area or NI role. Nor is someone in a given role required to have every skill indicated. For example, a quality improvement (QI) specialist is an NI role that would stress the *Analysis* functional area. An Informatics Nurse Specialist working in a quality improvement area would require competency in many of the indicated computer literacy skills including administration, communication, desktop, systems, and quality improvement, but would not likely need the simulation skills identified in the matrix. However, a quality assurance specialist, listed in the same functional area, would need knowledge and skills about simulations, especially if the NI in this role worked in an institution using simulation for staff development or for a vendor using this product.

The Functional Area-Competency Framework provides an example of the nursing informatics competencies for different functional areas within NI roles. Telehealth, which may be seen as more of an integrative area rather than a stand-alone functional role, is included to reflect intersections with various competencies. The list is not exhaustive, but presents beginning guidance to the essential NI competencies across computer literacy, information literacy, and professional development skills and knowledge. Currently the competencies are at different levels. In the future they may be re-evaluated, expanded, or collapsed.

Competencies and Metastructures

The components of metastructures—data, information, knowledge, and wisdom—can be compared to the elements in the competencies matrix. Using a patient care example, the beginning nurse uses skills that rely on the ability to obtain data. Computer skills, data entry, and the use of the patient's electronic medical record are the major focus of their practice. The experienced nurse builds on this and applies basic computer skills to information.

The INS has expertise in nursing, as well as higher levels of computer literacy, information literacy, and professional development and leadership. This increased level represents knowledge in nursing informatics. The INS analyzes systems and processes in order to apply knowledge to patient care, administration, research, or education. Last, the informatics innovator has achieved a level of knowledge coupled with experience, a combination that exemplifies wisdom. Wisdom in informatics may be the creation of unique methods for system design or evaluation, or the political finesse to justify purchase of a system.

The content in this appendix is not current and is of historical significance only.

Table 2. Informatics Competencies by NI Functional Areas

Competency Categories	Knowledge and Skills	Beginning Nurse	Experienced Nurse	Informatics Specialist	Informatics Innovator	Administration	Analysis	Compliance & Integrity Management	Consultation	Coordination, Facilitation, & Integration	Development	Education & Professional Development	Policy Development & Advocacy	Research & Evaluation	Integrated Areas
Computer Literacy															
	Computer Skills—Administration	X				X	X	X	X	X		X			X
	Computer Skills—Communication	X	X			X	X	X	X						X
	Computer Skills—Data Access	X													X
	Computer Skills—Documentation	X	X								X	X			X
	Computer Skills—Education	X	X									X			X
	Computer Skills—Monitoring	X	X	X						X	X	X	X		X
	Computer Skills—Basic Desktop Software	X	X	X		X	X		X	X	X	X			X
	Computer Skills—Systems		X	X		X	X	X	X			X	X	X	
	Computer Skills—Quality Improvement			X		X	X		X	X		X			X
	Computer Skills—Research		X			X			X	X	X	X		X	
	Computer Skills—Project Management			X	X					X	X	X		X	
	Computer Skills—Simulation					X	X	X	X	X	X	X	X	X	X
Information Literacy															
	Informatics Skills—Evaluation		X	X	X	X	X		X	X	X	X	X	X	X
	Informatics Skills—Role		X	X		X	X		X	X	X	X	X		
	Informatics Skills—System Maintenance		X	X		X	X		X	X	X	X	X		X
	Informatics Skills—Analysis			X	X	X	X		X	X	X	X	X	X	X
	Informatics Skills—Data/Data Structure			X		X	X	X	X	X	X	X	X	X	X
	Informatics Skills—Design & Development			X	X	X	X	X	X	X	X	X	X	X	X
	Informatics Skills—Fiscal Management			X	X	X	X		X	X	X	X	X	X	X
	Informatics Skills—Implementation			X		X	X		X	X	X	X			X
	Informatics Skills—Management			X	X	X	X	X	X			X	X	X	X
	Informatics Skills—Programming			X		X	X		X		X				
	Informatics Skills—Requirements			X		X	X	X	X	X	X	X	X	X	X

(continues)

The content in this appendix is not current and is of historical significance only.

Table 2. *Continued*

Competency Categories	Knowledge and Skills	Beginning Nurse	Experienced Nurse	Informatics Specialist	Informatics Innovator	Administration	Analysis	Compliance & Integrity Management	Consultation	Coordination, Facilitation, & Integration	Development	Education & Professional Development	Policy Development & Advocacy	Research & Evaluation	Integrated Areas
Information Literacy															
	Informatics Skills—System Selection			×		×	×	×	×	×	×		×	×	×
	Informatics Skills—Testing			×		×	×			×	×	×			×
	Informatics Skills—Training			×		×				×	×	×			×
	Informatics Knowledge—Impact	×	×	×	×	×	×	×	×	×	×	×	×	×	×
	Informatics Knowledge—Privacy/security	×	×	×		×	×	×	×	×	×	×	×	×	×
	Informatics Knowledge—Systems	×	×	×		×	×	×	×	×	×	×			×
	Informatics Knowledge—Research		×	×			×	×	×	×	×	×	×		×
	Informatics Knowledge—Regulations			×		×	×	×	×	×	×	×	×	×	×
	Informatics Knowledge—Usability/Human Factors			×	×	×	×		×	×	×	×	×	×	×
	Informatics Knowledge—Education			×	×	×	×		×	×	×	×		×	×
	Informatics Knowledge—Models & Theories			×	×	×	×	×	×	×	×	×	×	×	
	Informatics Knowledge—Nursing Classification, Taxonomies, & Nomenclature			×	×	×	×	×	×	×	×	×	×	×	×
	System Lifecycle			×										×	×
	Organization Change Management		×	×	×	×	×	×	×	×			×	×	×
	Systems Theory			×	×		×			×	×	×		×	×
	Management Science				×			×	×	×		×	×		×
	Standards for Privacy & Security	×	×	×	×	×	×	×	×	×	×	×	×	×	×
	Human Computer Interface			×	×		×			×	×	×		×	×
	Computer Assisted Instuction											×			
	Statistical Analysis			×	×	×	×				×			×	×
	Adapting information technology as a primary means of patient safety	×	×	×			×	×	×	×	×	×	×	×	×

The content in this appendix is not current and is of historical significance only.

Work in Progress

Work in NI competencies is evolving. There is no single consolidated list of competencies across educational levels, or a reference list of competencies for employers. Perhaps it is premature to cease all innovation, but the proliferation of lists can be confusing to the uninitiated.

In addition to numerous researchers, academics, and employers, many professional organizations are actively working toward identifying competencies for nursing informatics, such as:

- The American Medical Informatics Association (AMIA)'s 10x10 program (AMIA, 2006b).

- The AMIA Educational Workgroup.

- The HIMSS nursing informatics working group.

- An NLN Task Group on Informatics Competencies and subsequent initiatives (NLN, 2005a, 2005b).

- Technology Informatics Guiding Education Reform (TIGER, 2006).

NI Competencies: Conclusion

The work on informatics competencies has expanded greatly in the last five years. After the initial work of Staggers, et al (2001, 2002), numerous authors and agencies have now developed informatics competencies. The new competencies matrix (Table 2) matches competencies with typical NI functional areas. In the future, the rapid pace of technological change and generation of information and knowledge will present challenges for maintaining current and accurate competencies for nursing informatics. Faculty must understand competencies for nursing informatics to make NI an integral part of curricula and to stimulate research. Besides the educational arena, employers show a growing interest in competencies. More important, within the next few years, the multiple lists of NI competencies will benefit from consensus and consolidation.

References: NI Competencies

Alliance for Nursing Informatics (ANI). (2005). *Member organization report.* Retrieved October 10, 2007 from http://www.allianceni.org/doc/ANI_MemberOrgReport2005-06.pdf.

The content in this appendix is not current and is of historical significance only.

Androwich, I.M., Bickford, C.J., Button, P.J., Hunter, K.M., Murphy, J., & Sensmeier, J. (2003). *Clinical information systems: A framework for reaching the vision.* Washington, DC: American Nurses Publishing.

American Library Association (ALA). (2006). *Information literacy competency standards for higher education.* Retrieved October 10, 2007 from http://www.ala.org/acrl/ilcomstan.html.

American Medical Informatics Association (AMIA). (2006b). *Oregon health & science university biomedical informatics distance learning course.* Retrieved October 10, 2007 from http://www.amia.org/10x10/partners/ohsu.

American Nurses Credentialing Center (ANCC). (2007). *Informatics Nurse Certification.* Retrieved October 10, 2007 from http://www.nursecredentialing.org/ancc/cert/eligibility/informatics.html.

Barton, A.J. (2005). Cultivating informatics competencies in a community of practice. *Nursing Administration Quarterly, 29*(4), 323–328.

Curran, C.R. (2003). Informatics competencies for nurse practitioners. *American Association of Critical Care Nurses Clinical Issues, 14*(3), 320–330.

Desjardins, K.S., Cook, S.S., Jenkins, M., & Bakken, S. (2005). Effect of an informatics for evidence-based practice curriculum on nursing informatics competencies. *International Journal of Medical Informatics, 74*(11–12), 1012–1020.

Garde, S., Harrison, D., & Hovenga, E. (2005). Skill needs for nurses in their role as health informatics professionals: A survey in the context of global health informatics education. *International Journal of Medical Informatics, 74*(11–12), 899–907.

Healthcare Information and Management Systems Society (HIMSS). (2005). *HLA competency directory: ensuring future leaders meet the challenges of managing the nation's healthcare organizations.* Retrieved October 10, 2007 from http://www.himss.org/asp/ContentRedirector.asp?ContentId=65250.

The content in this appendix is not current and is of historical significance only.

Healthcare Leadership Alliance (HLA). (2005). *Competency directory*. Retrieved October 10, 2007 from http://www.healthcare leadership alliance.org/directory.htm.

Institute of Medicine (IOM). (2003). *Health professions education: A bridge to quality.* Washington, DC: National Academies Press.

Jiang, W., Chen, W., & Chen, Y. (2004). Important computer competencies for the nursing profession. *Journal of Nursing Research, 12*(3), 213–225.

Marin, H.F. (2005). Nursing informatics: Current issues around the world. *International Journal of Medical Informatics, 74,* 857–860.

McNeil, B.J., Elfrink, V.L., Pierce, S.T., Beyea, S.C., Bickford, C.J., & Averill, C. (2005). Nursing informatics knowledge and competencies: A national survey of nursing education programs in the United States. *International Journal of Medical Informatics, 74*(11–12), 1021–1030.

McNeil, B.J., & Odom, S.K. (2000). Nursing informatics education in the United States: Proposed undergraduate curriculum. *Health Informatics Journal, 6,* 32–38.

National League for Nursing (NLN). (2005a). *Core competencies of nurse educators with task statements.* Retrieved October 10, 2007 from http://www.nln.org/profdev/corecompetencies.pdf.

National League for Nursing (NLN). (2005b). *Task group on informatics competencies.* Retrieved December 4, 2006 from http://www.nln.org/aboutnln/AdvisoryCouncils_TaskGroups/informatics.htm

Saranto, K., & Leino-Kilpi, H. (1997). Computer literacy in nursing; developing the information technology syllabus in nursing education. *Journal of Advanced Nursing, 25,* 377–385.

Staggers, N., & Gassert, C. (2000). Competencies for nursing informatics. In B. Carty (Ed.), *Nursing informatics: Education for practice* (pp. 17–34). New York: Springer-Verlag.

The content in this appendix is not current and is of historical significance only.

Staggers, N., Gassert, C., & Curran, C. (2001). Informatics competencies for nurses at four levels of practice. *Journal of Nursing Education, 4*(7), 303–316.

Staggers, N., Gassert, C., & Curran, C. (2002). A Delphi study to determine informatics competencies for nurses at four levels of practice. *Nursing Research, 51*(6), 383–390.

Technology Informatics Guiding Educational Reform (TIGER). (2006). *TIGER Summit.* Retrieved October 10, 2007 from http://www.tigersummit.com/

The Integration of Nursing Informatics

As the use of technology increasingly becomes integrated into nursing and every nursing role, the boundaries between the roles of nurses and informatics nurses are becoming even more blurred. It becomes important to identify the commonalities along the practice continuum for nurses in all levels and specialties, and also the functions that make the practice of nursing informatics unique among nursing specialties. Information is central to healthcare delivery. All nurses must be skilled in managing and communicating information and are primarily concerned with the content of that information, but nursing informatics is especially concerned with the creation, structure, and delivery of that information: from the use of technology at the bedside to provide direct care, to giving the healthcare consumer point-of-need access to healthcare information, through exploiting the data underlying this information to create new nursing knowledge. This range in the use of information and technology can be visualized on a continuum as seen in Figure 4.

Figure 4. A Continuum of Integrating Information and Technology into Nursing Practice.

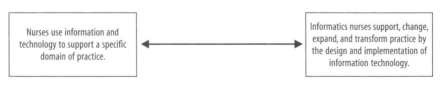

The content in this appendix is not current and is of historical significance only.

Nursing informatics is also integrated into other healthcare informatics specialties. The INS is often responsible for implementing or coordinating projects involving multiple disciplines. The INS is expected to interact with professionals involved in all phases of the information systems lifecycle and with professionals in all aspects of system utilization. NI can be conceptualized either as an integral part of healthcare informatics or as a specialty within healthcare informatics. Core concepts are common to multiple informatics disciplines. There are also individual concepts and methods that are unique to one discipline. Two concept diagrams from Englebardt and Nelson (2002) demonstrate the different views of the role of NI in relation to other healthcare informatics specialties (see Figure 5).

NI is also integrated into all aspects of the healthcare continuum. This integration provides access to healthcare information at the point of need, such as at the bedside in acute healthcare settings, ambulatory care settings, at home, or even when traveling locally or globally.

Figure 5. The Healthcare Informatics Specialist: Two Models

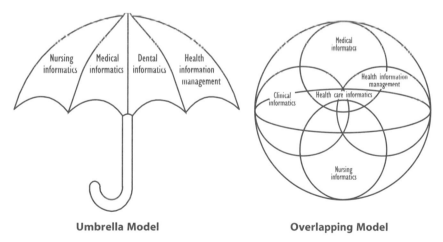

Umbrella Model　　　　　**Overlapping Model**

Reprinted with permission (Englebardt & Nelson, 2002)

The content in this appendix is not current and is of historical significance only.

The Boundaries of Nursing Informatics

This section summarizes the differences between NI and other specialties in nursing, and between NI and other informatics specialties. To reiterate, NI is a specialty that integrates nursing science, computer science, and information science to manage and communicate data, information, knowledge, and wisdom in nursing practice. Critical thinking is a requirement of all nursing practice, and NI facilitates this critical thinking through the integration of data, information, knowledge, and wisdom to support patients, nurses, and other practitioners in their decision-making in all roles and settings. The difference between NI and other nursing specialties is the emphasis on informatics concepts, tools, and methods to facilitate nursing practice.

Although some outside the specialty might consider NI synonymous with information technology, technology alone does not define NI. The synthesis of data and information into knowledge and wisdom is central to NI, and information technology merely supports this process. INSs have adopted the anticipatory proactive stance characterized by Hannah, Ball, and Edwards (1994), and continuously strive to exploit technology in the design, structure, and presentation of information. They also consider the impact on healthcare delivery in general, and the nursing process specifically. Figure 6 illustrates the connection between the different foci of nursing and NI. These occur along a continuum without distinct boundaries.

Figure 6. Nursing and Nursing Informatics Foci

Nursing Focus	Nursing Informatics Focus
Nurses, patients, health, environment	→ Information user, information recipients, information exchange
Content of information, support for evidence-based practice changes	→ Design, structure, and representation of data as information
Using information applications and technology	→ Develop, implement, and evaluate applications and technology, ensuring the quality, effectiveness, efficiency, and usability of applications and technology

The content in this appendix is not current and is of historical significance only.

NI is also differentiated from other informatics specialties. Each informatics specialty is aligned uniquely with its primary role, requiring that INSs augment their base of nursing knowledge with unique informatics skills. Nursing informatics is recognized both as a component of the broad field of healthcare informatics and as a specialty within nursing (Brennan, 2002). This results in a unique body of knowledge and demonstrates the need for advanced preparation unique to nursing. NI incorporates informatics concepts used by others, but applies them to a foundation of nursing. What differentiates an INS or an IN from other informatics specialists is the knowledge of nursing content and process. The synthesis of informatics and nursing results in an integrated whole that is greater than its parts. Thus, an understanding of how informatics can support patient care in the context of the nursing process is fundamental to NI. Core components of informatics knowledge and skills underpin all informatics specialties, such as the use of technology, computer literacy, and data management structures. There are also components unique to each discipline such as their taxonomy.

Tenets of Nursing Informatics

- Nursing informatics contains a unique body of knowledge, preparation, and experience, and uses identifiable techniques and methods.

- Nursing informatics supports the clinical and non-clinical efforts of nurses and other providers to improve the quality of care and the welfare of healthcare consumers. Information or informatics methods alone do not improve patient care; rather, this information is used by clinicians and managers to improve care, information management, and patient outcomes.

- Nursing informatics collaborates with and is closely linked to other health-related informatics specialties.

- Although concerned with information technology, nursing informatics focuses on efficient and effective delivery of complete and accurate information in order to achieve quality outcomes.

- Human factors, human–computer interaction, ergonomics, and usability concepts are interwoven throughout the practice of NI.

- Nursing informatics promotes established, emerging, and innovative information technologies.

The content in this appendix is not current and is of historical significance only.

- The key ethical concerns of nursing informatics include advocating privacy and ensuring the confidentiality and security of healthcare data and information.

Ethics in Nursing Informatics

Nursing has a long history of applying ethical principles to nursing practice, with a primary concern for the patient and a commitment to the professional code of ethics for nurses. *Code of Ethics for Nurses with Interpretive Statements* (ANA, 2001) serves as a guide for the informatics nurse facing ethical issues, dilemmas, and decisions. The ANA policy on privacy and confidentiality (ANA, 2006b) addresses HIPAA legislation and the ethics of protecting information in a changing healthcare environment. Additionally, with the increase in electronic health records (EHRs) across multiple systems, decisions related to the use of information in the EHR must strike a balance between "ethically justified ends and otherwise appropriate means" (IMIA, 2006). The primacy of concern for patients and the commitment to this code of nursing ethics form a foundation for considering ethical issues in nursing, including nursing informatics. However, the practice of nursing informatics, a highly specialized and non-traditional nursing practice, also needs its own specialty-specific ethical guidelines.

Ethical questions often arise when common corporate business practices conflict with the ethical mandates of healthcare professionals. The INS brings an integrated, systems perspective to discussions of ethical issues, such as:

- Is a code of ethics integrated into the expanding distributed environment of electronic health information and healthcare service delivery?

- Is the individual responding to a healthcare related e-mail or web site inquiry appropriately licensed and qualified?

- In healthcare-related electronic communication, are appropriate safeguards in place to protect the sender's identity and privacy, the content and integrity of messages, and the respondent's identity?

The International Medical Informatics Association (IMIA) has published a detailed code of ethics for health information professionals. The IMIA code is meant to guide decision-making for "gathering, processing, storing, communicating, using, manipulating, and accessing health information" (IMIA, 2006). It offers ethical guidance uniquely applicable to nursing informatics. Among its general principles, two are of special interest to nursing informatics: information privacy and disposition, and legitimate infringement. The principle of information privacy and disposition states that all persons have a fundamental right to privacy, and hence control over the collection, storage, access, use, communication, manipulation, and disposition of data about themselves. However, the principle of legitimate infringement states that this fundamental right is tempered by the legitimate, appropriate, and relevant data needs of a free, responsible, and democratic society, and by the equal and competing rights of other persons.

Furthermore, INSs should understand and apply the basic principles of autonomy, beneficence, non-malfeasance, and justice as they relate to the practice of informatics (ANA, 2001). The INS encounters questions of biomedical ethics throughout systems development, implementation, and administration. For example, informatics professionals including nurse specialists must determine whether patients see all of their lab results online, perhaps before a clinician has seen them. This decision may be less a technical question than an ethical one concerning the principle of patient autonomy. Security standards respond to the principles of autonomy and non-malfeasance. In the United States, decisions concerning the appropriate access and use of data may be guided by both HIPAA rules and the ethical principle of justice.

The general principles described by the IMIA and ANA codes provide a solid ethical foundation for INSs. The INS has a responsibility to advocate for data confidentiality, integrity, and security, quality management of information, and legitimate data use. These needs must be balanced with users' timely access to accurate data for decision-making in all settings. The role of ethics in informatics practice is expanding, and INSs are in a unique position to make or share in decisions of informatics policy and operations. INSs can reconcile organizational risk with users' needs for timely data access. They can serve as the voice of wisdom—as translators and advocates for users who also understand the relevant ethical, political, and technological considerations.

New computing approaches such as knowledge discovery, clinical data repositories (CDR), and data warehouses have already created new opportunities for the INS to apply ethical principles. Vast electronic stores of digitized personal data already exist. Contemporary organizations are grappling with complex issues like regulation of data access

The content in this appendix is not current and is of historical significance only.

such that only appropriate data is visible only to appropriate users. As technologies evolve and data stores increase, the ethics of data use and protection will become increasingly intricate, requiring continual evaluation and monitoring. Informatics professionals must consider the following ethical responsibilities (IMIA, 2006):

- To ensure personal competence, integrity, diligence, and responsibility for all actions performed.

- To ensure that an electronic record, or the data contained in it, are used only for the stated purposes for which the data was collected or for purposes that are otherwise ethically defensible.

- To ensure that appropriate structures are in place to evaluate the technical, legal, and ethical acceptability of the data collection, storage, retrieval, processing, accessing, communication, and utilization of data in the settings in which they carry out their work.

- To ensure that healthcare professionals are informed about the status of the information services upon which users rely and must immediately advise users of any problems or difficulties that might be associated with or could reasonably be expected to arise in connection with these informatics services (IMIA 2006, p 6). (For example, processes such as phone trees for notification of system difficulties need to be addressed in both the planning and implementation of those services.)

In conclusion, the INS has the opportunity and responsibility to face the ethical ramifications of design, implementation, and utilization of healthcare information systems and data obtained through reporting mechanisms. The INS is challenged to balance the improvement of health care with individual privacy, security, and safety. Balancing the autonomy of patients and their health information against the just use of health information to benefit others requires thoughtful consideration across multiple levels. Given the complexity and challenge of making ethical decisions related to healthcare information systems, the INS must contribute to and act in accordance with a general understanding of the applicable ethical principles.

The Future of Nursing Informatics

Our discipline is rapidly changing: it will change even while this document is being printed. Three trends will likely influence the direction of this change: positions and competencies for nurses and informatics, technological aspects of the field, and changes in healthcare delivery and regulatory requirements.

Trends in Positions and Competencies for Nurses and Informatics

The boundaries between INSs, other nurses, and associated health informatics disciplines are blurring. As information and technology are further integrated into the workplace, nurses in all settings will gain informatics knowledge and skills. The number and complexity of informatics competencies for nurses will continue to escalate. Some informatics competencies ascribed to informatics specialists will likely transfer to mainstream nurses, and the level of competencies required for INSs will continue to expand. Thus, the baseline set of NI competencies required of nurses at all levels will rise.

In the last few years, new areas of nursing have been incorporated into nursing informatics. For example, nurses who heavily use information and technology, such as telehealth nurses, may be considered one type of IN. As others in nursing design, implement, and evaluate informatics solutions, the scope of nursing informatics will expand still more. Nursing informatics is becoming a world community with fewer distinctions and more commonalities among INSs everywhere.

The role boundaries between other health informatics roles and NI are less conspicuous than in the past. One of the centerpieces of NI practice is its cross-disciplinary nature, with INSs often leading cross-disciplinary projects to craft usable informatics solutions for use by many disciplines. INSs have assumed executive positions in the health informatics arena. INSs and their health informatics colleagues serve in many of the same positions, blurring boundaries while using a shared set of functions, skills, and knowledge. This trend will likely continue as professional informatics organizations define a shared set of core knowledge and skills required by all informatics specialties. Probably the clearest trend is evolving change in the functional areas for INSs, a continual move from a generic set of skills for any one discipline toward a shared set of competencies based on functional areas required to enact a particular position (i.e., clinical analyst, informatics executive, futurist, KDD researcher, or database developer).

Trends in Technology

Information technology is becoming commonplace in our daily lives as well as in health care. For the first time in history, a generation exists never having known a world without the Internet, cell phones, online social networks, blogs, and other electronic media. People raised on this technology will be entering the healthcare field as knowledge workers as well as consumers of healthcare delivery. Implications for NI are:

- New models of work and education for technologically sophisticated users who are less resistant to technology and in fact demand it.

- Adapting to users with less skill in face-to-face communications.

- Consumers with even greater expectations of accelerated information and technology implementation.

Several advances in technology will likely impact nursing informatics in the future. A number of these are outlined in the following sections.

Nanotechnology

Nanotechnology—microscopic technology on the order of one-billionth of a meter—will likely impact the diagnosis and treatment of many diseases and conditions (Gordon, Lutz, Boninger & Cooper, 2007). Some of the pending technologies that will affect INSs, clinicians, and patients may include:

- New methods for medication administration
  - Sensing patient's internal drug levels with miniature medical diagnostic tools circulating in patients' bloodstreams.
  - Chemotherapy delivered directly to a tumor site, reducing systemic side-effects.

- New monitoring devices for the home:
  - A talking pill bottle that lets patients push a button to hear prescription information.
  - Bathroom counters that announce whether it is safe to mix two medications.
  - A shower with built-in scales to calculate body mass index (Hong Kong Polytechnic University).

- Measuring devices in the bathroom to track urine frequency and output and upload these data to a system or care manager.

- Non-invasive blood glucose monitors to eliminate sticks; sensors to compute blood. sugar levels using a multi-wavelength reflective dispersion photometer (Hong Kong Polytechnic University).

Tools for managing public health concerns

The threat of terrorism and bioterrorism, and the need for improved disease management across traditional boundaries, drive the demand for new tools and solutions that will concern the INS. Partnership with public health professionals and the emergence of public health informatics is a response to the need for population management tools and early disease detection.

Devices and hardware

The increased miniaturization of devices will change where and how IT solutions will be deployed. No perfect hardware solution exists in the market today to address all diverse nursing workflows and mobile caregiver demands. An emphasis on ergonomics and human-computer interaction will lead to new solutions to support diverse workflow requirements.

New integrated technologies—cell phones, smart phones, PDA's, and multi-functional devices—will increase common access to health information. These solutions are becoming ubiquitous in daily life. They will change clinicians' and patients' expectations and their interactions with technology. In particular, providers will be challenged to know as much about new disease treatments and research findings as patients with these devices are.

Wearable computing

Wearable computing is a revolutionary paradigm that shatters myths about what computers are and how they should be used. A computer can be worn, much as eyeglasses or clothing are worn, and interactions with the user based on the context of the situation. With heads-up displays, embedded sensors in fabrics, unobtrusive input devices, personal wireless local area networks, and a host of other context sensing and

The content in this appendix is not current and is of historical significance only.

communication tools, wearable computers can act as intelligent assistants or data collection and analysis devices.

Many of these devices are available now. Smart fabrics with embedded sensors have been on the commercial market since 2000 and are being used in shirts, gloves, and other clothing. These wearable computer and remote monitoring systems are intertwined with the user's activity so that the technology becomes transparent. Sensors and devices can gather data during the patient's daily routine, providing healthcare providers or researchers periodic or continuous data on the subject's health at work, school, exercise, and sleep, rather than the current snapshot captured during a typical hospital or clinic visit. A few applications for wearable computing include (OSNF, 2007):

- Sudden Infant Death Syndrome monitoring for infants
- Ambulatory cardiac and respiratory monitoring
- Monitoring of ventilation during exercise
- Monitoring rescue worker's vital signs
- Activity level of post-stroke patients
- Patterns of breathing in asthma
- Assessment of stress in individuals
- Arrhythmia detection and control of selected cardiac conditions
- Daily activity monitors
- Monitoring heat stress and dehydration

Wearable computing is applicable to workers as well as consumers or patients:

- Proximity badges and RFID (radio frequency identification) to track providers for workflow or allow log on to systems.
- Glasses with a heads-up display of vital signs or images without losing focus on the patient (MIT Media Lab, 2007).
- Bar code scanners that fit on a finger, or wrist-activated input devices.

Future developments for input methods may also apply to the healthcare market. For example, an "interface-free," touch-driven computer screen, manipulated intuitively with the fingertips, responds to varying

The content in this appendix is not current and is of historical significance only.

levels of pressure. Another example is virtual keyboards using Bluetooth technology, in which a keyboard can be displayed and used on any surface (*ThinkGeek*, 2007).

Robotics

The use of robotics in patient care will expand. Robots have been used for many years to deliver supplies to patient care areas. Robotics enable remote surgeries and virtual reality surgical procedures. At Johns Hopkins, robots are being used as translators for patients (Greenback, 2007). Hand-assist devices help patients regain strength after a stroke (*Science Daily*, 2007). Robots are providing a remote presence to allow physicians to virtually examine patients by manipulating remote cameras (Cisco Systems, 2007). In the future, robots may also be used in direct patient care, for instance, to help lift morbidly obese patients.

Knowledge representation

As more and more electronic data become available for and about patients over their lifetime, clinicians will need advanced tools to help lo cate and synthesize this vast volume of data. New research will yield advances in displaying vast amounts of data to clinicians to optimize patient care and patient and clinician efficiencies while avoiding medical errors. NI may need more nurses trained in knowledge representation, semantic representation, and other knowledge areas. This also has implications for knowledge discovery in databases, data quality, and a continued emphasis on data standards and data quality

Nurses constantly make complex and diverse decisions in their daily practice. Decision-making must consider relevant evidence-based and patient-specific information. As nurse decision-making becomes more complex, the need for computerized clinical decision support will increase. In the absence of explicit evidence-based guidelines for nursing decisions, novel technologies will be necessary to synthesize evidence from the literature or induce models from clinical data. Knowledge discovery in databases could play an important role in the induction of clinical knowledge models.

Genomics

Advances in mapping the human genome and understanding individual DNA will have a dramatic impact on what we know about pa-

The content in this appendix is not current and is of historical significance only.

tients. These data, especially once they are integrated into EHRs or personal health records (PHRs), will lead to advances in customized patient care and customized medications targeted to individual responses to medications. Care and medication can be precisely customized to patients based on their unique DNA profile and how they have responded to medications and other interventions in the past. This will dramatically change how patients are managed for specific diseases and conditions, and extend into the prevention of some diseases.

The inherent complexity of customized patient care will demand computerized clinical decision support. Predictive disease models based on patients' DNA profiles will emerge as clinicians better understand DNA mapping. These advances have implications for a new model of care and for the INS's participation in the development of genomic IT solutions. More than ever, patients will need to be partners in this development. Genomics will lead to many specialized advances in care delivery and be linked to exact, individualized data within a personal health record (PHR). Subsequently, advanced disease management with the ultimate goal of disease prevention will be possible. This change has many implications for ethics as well as informatics. In fact, genomics competencies and curricular guidelines are available online (ANA, 2007)..

Educational technologies

Evolving teaching technologies are changing the education techniques used in the classroom, the lab, and the clinical setting. For example, patient care simulators allow students to run programmed care scenarios in a safe environment and provide innovative options for teaching critical thinking skills. Group learning tools such as clickers, used in interactive teaching, can change how students engage with class content as well as how they learn to function as members of a team (Michaelsen, Fink, & Knight, 2007). Distance education technologies such as web-based course management systems and the related student support services are challenging basic education concepts such as what academic resources must be included in a library collection or how a university defines a credit hour of education. Administrative information systems are automating basic university functions like admissions, registration, student record management, grant management, and financial aid, for example (Nelson et al., 2006). This automation is forcing institutions to review and in many cases to revise their educational policies and procedures. These technologies require a paradigm shift in

The content in this appendix is not current and is of historical significance only.

knowledge delivery, which affects students, instructors, and course content.

In these modern educational settings, faculty, with little more than office applications for support, continue to manage large amounts of data about individual students, curricula, and accreditation. Comprehensive, enterprise-wide educational information systems that integrate administrative and academic functions are just beginning to provide educators with tools to manage all aspects of the educator role. As nursing informatics faculty become actively involved in the design, monitoring, and evaluation of these comprehensive systems, they will create the healthcare educational institutions of the future.

Traditional tuition models are a barrier to the globalization of education, but they are being slowly eroded. New educational models are already being created as universities reach students beyond their walls or create virtual educational experiences, e.g., partnering with other institutions to deliver classes to students across a region. Perhaps in the future, universities will partner with business entities and vendors to create other innovative models of education.

Curriculum design will change. Information is now generated and made available so quickly that baseline knowledge for students will evolve away from specific content to methods of finding accurate, current information and knowledge. Future students may not be evaluated on specific knowledge for one area or course, but instead be evaluated on their growth over time. The INS will be at the center of this union of informatics and new educational models because of its focus on managing information.

Tools for patient access to health information

Patients will continue to become stronger partners with providers, with increased accountability for their own care. This type of model will require solutions and patient education by clinical nurses and INSs to devise the best methods of care as well as solutions to monitor and maintain patients' health.

Expanded use of IT in nursing

Technology use will increase everywhere in our work and home settings, perhaps even constantly traveling with us as wearable devices. Two implications are outlined here.

The content in this appendix is not current and is of historical significance only.

One is a current concern about students relying on available, structured information, computerized alerts, and reminders in systems such as EHRs and DSSs. Some educators and administrators now are concerned that if students rely on available, structured information, computerized alerts, and reminders in systems such as EHRs and DSSs, their critical thinking skills may diminish. Future INSs and educators will determine and test new academic and practice models. Perhaps academic applications will be designed differently than practice applications designed to encourage questioning and active cognitive engagement. Or system designers may need to modify systems to promote a different cognitive engagement by practitioners. Or educators may teach a new level of human information processing to maximize human capabilities, one beyond students needing to memorize structures for a physical examination and similar static information stored in an EHR. In this model, information technology serves as an aid to, not a replacement for, human thinking and judgment.

Reliability is the other implication of the increasing pervasiveness of IT. As applications are increasingly integrated into healthcare, the impact of downtime becomes more severe and quick recovery methods imperative. Especially with order management in place, institutions must ensure continuous business operations with uninterrupted access to applications and data. Strategies and technologies to support continuous uptime are available, and the INS is typically involved in defining, designing, and installing them. Pervasive computing creates a new standard for information access even when there is no power supply, like a laptop powered by a hand crank (OLPC, 2007). Thus, INSs must be strong advocates for systems to be continuously available. Likewise, they can be intimately involved in disaster recovery, including being an advocate for funding allocations for recovery methods.

In 2005, Hurricane Katrina emphasized the importance of redundant systems and effective disaster recovery procedures. Requirements for current and future systems will focus on prevention rather include reaction as well as these features:

- 24×7 operation and performance with redundancies throughout the system, failovers, and tested high reliability.

- Tools to assist in monitoring and managing the IT environment, monitor system use, and identify technology issues before system failure occurs.

The content in this appendix is not current and is of historical significance only.

- Scalable IT solutions as more clinical applications come online.
- Solutions that IT departments can manage without in-depth technology expertise.

Implications for INSs

INSs will need to have a systematic method for becoming aware of emerging technologies and their projected impact(s) to healthcare and informatics. INSs can be essential leaders and partners for the safe and intelligent incorporation of new technology and techniques into health informatics solutions. The content or information on devices is still the most critical component, and INSs can serve as content designers. Areas such as genomics may have ethical ramifications, and INSs must ensure that they are respected. Sub-specialization within NI will continue, and INSs may find themselves specializing in the safe use of particular technologies.

All of these areas have implications for curricular design and education. The expansion of technology amplifies the need for continuous availability of systems. On the other hand, the "digital divide" in large remains: a significant number of people have little access to information technology. INSs can also take the lead in eliminating the digital divide between those with access to information and those without. In all situations, INSs can advocate and apply methods for users to learn and use new technologies effectively and safely.

Trends in Healthcare Delivery and Regulation

One force that has driven information technology and EHR installations in the United States is a national emphasis on patient safety, including technology installation as a focal point for reducing errors in healthcare. Also responsible is the fact that health organizations such as AHRQ and IHI, as well as non-health organizations like Leapfrog, are impatient with slow progress, to the point that they are providing incentives for health institutions to implement informatics solutions. Other forces will likely escalate the pace of adoption. Organizations are using value-versus-return-on-investment models to justify health IT and pay-for-performance models will likely accelerate EHR installations. Data are becoming more visible to consumers and hospital boards. Organizations will continue to increase the transparency of data and, more importantly, improve the care being delivered.

The content in this appendix is not current and is of historical significance only.

Regulatory requirements and standards will shape the future. INSs will be involved in defining these and future standards, and in designing, building, implementing, using, and certifying products that comply. A number of projects are underway, among them:

- Certification Commission for Healthcare Information Technology (CCHIT). "CCHIT is a recognized certification body (RCB) for electronic health records and their networks, and an independent, voluntary, private-sector initiative." Their mission is "to accelerate the adoption of health information technology by creating an efficient, credible, and sustainable product certification program." (CCHIT, 2007)

- HL7 is defining interoperability standards for systems.

- The IEEEP2407 working group is developing standards for personalized health informatics.

- The Joint Commission continues to expand regulatory compliance for patient safety, e.g., national patient safety goals, medication reconciliation, and other requirements with implications for the INS.

- The Health Information Technology Standards Panel (HITSP) is harmonizing industry-wide health IT standards.

- The Nationwide Health Information Network (NHIN) initiative is creating prototype architectures for widespread health information exchange.

- The FDA (Food and Drug Administration) has several initiatives underway:
  - Bar code label requirements for human drug products and biological products (FDA, 2007a).
  - Draft guidelines for the safe and effective use of radio frequency devices.
  - Nanotechnology development (FDA, 2007b) and potential expansion of products covered, e.g., advanced decision support tools and similar informatics applications.

Care delivery models

Care is no longer a local phenomenon. Patients in rural ICUs can be monitored remotely by intensivists and ICU nurses. Pharmacists can provide remote pharmacological assistance to rural areas. Radiologists

The content in this appendix is not current and is of historical significance only.

can read images in real time from anywhere in the world. Physicians are assisted by robots as they examine patients in distant locations.

Care is no longer limited to traditional healthcare settings, even when it is delivered locally. Clinicians are now available in retail stores, work settings, and other non-traditional places. These new settings will require new design, deployment, and support models that will challenge the NI specialist. INS involvement in the development of the robust health information infrastructure includes but is not limited to:

- Continued innovation of systems and expansion into less traditional settings such as long-term care and rural communities

- Personal health records will become more numerous. INSs will increasingly advocate for and assist patients with developing such individually maintained records. These can include one's own electronic vaccination history, past medical history, medications, allergies, condition, status, and visit history in an easily accessible online format. Patients' online communication with healthcare providers will continue to increase, as well.

- Clinical data repositories and regional health information organizations will support accurate, timely, and secure transfer of patient data across care settings (ultimately across hospitals, clinics, pharmacies, laboratories, clinician office, long-term care facilities, and others).

Consumer informatics

Patients will become stronger partners with providers, with increased accountability for their own care and greater interest in access to their own EMR data. As consumers become more technically adept, they will consider their electronic healthcare data as necessary and accessible as their online banking information or stock transactions. Likewise, consumers will begin monitoring and managing the health of younger *and* older family members for whom they are responsible.

External partnerships

Healthcare will likely see non-traditional organizations entering the healthcare arena. For example, one company with an online application for individual, secure financial records is now investigating expansion into personal health records. Likewise, healthcare should create new, non-traditional partnerships. Perhaps a partnership with the video-gaming industry would also be fruitful for interactive EHRs and yield ideas for optimal user interfaces.

Implications for INSs

New care models have vast implications for informatics nurses. These new delivery models will require INSs to continue developing informatics solutions for care in multiple, remote locations. INSs should have a key role in informatics solutions that emphasize quality care (McCormick et al., 2007). We need new models to shorten the time from design to installation in the systems life cycle. An 18- to 24-month build and implementation cycle is not tenable in an era of rapidly changing technology, care delivery, and expanding information access.

With the increasing number of information technology installations and the need to respond to burgeoning regulatory requirements, INSs will be at centerstage for all phases of the systems lifecycle. They will be developing and implementing new informatics solutions, ensuring data quality for implemented solutions, and evaluating the impact of solutions. The new model of consumer informatics will require technical solutions and patient education jointly from clinical nurses and INSs. INSs will need to devise the best methods of care as well as designing solutions that enable patients to monitor and maintain their own health. INSs will play a key role in designing new tools for data capture and analyses to comply with regulatory guidelines.

NI Future and Trends: Conclusions

The positions and competencies of nurses, changes in technology, and new trends in health delivery and regulation will shape the future of nursing informatics. Important concepts underlying these trends:

- Preparing for and evolving with new information and technology changes.

- Inventing and delivering new educational models to teach both new and existing nursing professionals.

The content in this appendix is not current and is of historical significance only.

- Designing, developing, implementing, and evaluating solutions for new information technologies across all areas of nursing and health settings.

- Incorporating newer technologies and methods to redesign care, research and administrative processes.

- Pioneering, designing, and facilitating changes in care models as they evolve away from episodic care toward more predictive and preventive models.

- Focusing on usability—designing and evaluating how information is presented to promote ease of use and adoption (human–computer interaction).

The global nature of informatics is already clear. In the future, care models and data will be shared even more widely. New technologies will create wider access to information and the need for a new generation of data and information management skills, analytic tools, new educational models, and different cognitive skills. Traditional boundaries of institutions, care delivery, and education will continue to erode. New positions and functional areas are emerging. Increased collaboration among NI colleagues and a shared scope and standard of NI practice will be the hallmark of the future.

References: Future and Trends

Certification Commission for Healthcare Information Technology (CCHIT). (2007). Home page. Retrieved October 10, 2007 from http://www.cchit.org/

Cisco Systems. (2007). Telemedicine pioneer helps physicians on the move stay close to patients. Retrieved October 10, 2007 from http://www.cisco.com/application/pdf/en/us/guest/netsol/ns554/c647/cdccont_0900aecd804073a3.pdf

Food and Drug Administration (FDA). (2007a). *FDA rule requires bar codes on drugs and blood to help reduce errors.* Retrieved October 10, 2007 from http://www.fda.gov/oc/initiatives/barcode-sadr/

Food and Drug Administration (FDA). (2007b). *FDA nanotechnology task force report.* Retrieved October 10, 2007 from www.fda.gov/nanotechnology.

The content in this appendix is not current and is of historical significance only.

Gordon, A.T., Lutz, G.E., Boninger, M.L., & Cooper, R.A. (2007). Introduction to nanotechnology: potential applications in physical medicine and rehabilitation. *American Journal of Physical Medicine & Rehabilitation*, *86*(3), 225– 241.

Greenback, L. (2007). Robot aids Johns Hopkins patients. *The Baltimore Examiner*. Retrieved January 9, 2007 from http://www.examiner.com/a-498079~Robot_aids_Johns_Hopkins_patients.html.

McCormick, K.A., Delaney, C.J., Brennan, P.F., Effken, J.A., Kendrick, K., Murphy, J., et al. (2007). Guideposts to the future—An agenda for nursing informatics. *Journal of the American Medical Informatics Association*, *14*(1), 19–24.

Massachusetts Institute of Technology (MIT) Media Lab. (2007). *Wearable computing*. Retrieved October 10, 2007 from http://www.media.mit.edu/wearables.

Michaelsen, M., Fink, L, & Knight, A. (2007) Team based learning: The power of teams for powerful learning. Retrieved October 10, 2007 from http://www.ou.edu/idp/teamlearning/

Nelson, R., & Ball, M. (Eds.). (2004) *Consumer informatics: Applications and strategies in cyber healthcare*. New York: Springer Verlag.

Nelson, R., Meyer, L., Rizzolo, M.A., Rutar, P., Proto, M.B., & Newbold, S. (2006). The evolution of educational information systems and nurse faculty roles. *Nursing Education Perspectives*. *27*(5), 189–195.

Offray Specialty Narrow Fabrics (OSNF). (2007). *Smart textiles*. Retrieved October 10, 2007 from http://www.osnf.com/p_smart.html

One Laptop per Child (OLPC). (2007). *A $100 laptop for the world's children's education*. Retrieved October 10, 2007 from http://www.laptop.org/

Science Daily. (2007). *Robotic brace aids stroke recovery*. Retrieved October 10, 2007 from http://www.sciencedaily.com/releases/2007/03/070321105223.htm

The content in this appendix is not current and is of historical significance only.

ThinkGeek. (2007). *Bluetooth Laser Virtual Keyboard*. Retrieved October 10, 2007 from http://www.thinkgeek.com/computing/input/8193/

Mendelson, H. (2005). *Moore's law*. Retrieved October 10, 2007 from http://www.thocp.net/biographies/papers/moores_law.htm

The content in this appendix is not current and is of historical significance only.

STANDARDS OF NURSING INFORMATICS PRACTICE

Nursing informatics (NI) is the specialty that integrates nursing science, computer science, and information science to manage and communicate data, information, knowledge, and wisdom in nursing practice. Nursing informatics facilitates the integration of data, information, knowledge, and wisdom to support patients, nurses, and other providers in their decision-making in all roles and settings. This support is accomplished through the use of information structures, information processes, and information technology.

The goal of nursing informatics is to improve the health of populations, communities, families, and individuals by optimizing information management and communication. These activities include the design and use of informatics solutions and technology to support all areas of nursing, including, but not limited to, the direct provision of care, establishing effective administrative systems, managing and delivering educational experiences, enhancing lifelong learning, and supporting nursing research.

The standards of nursing informatics practice include two components: standards of practice and standards of professional performance. Each standard includes measurement criteria that provide more detail about the expected knowledge, skills, and abilities necessary to meet that standard. Some standards include additional measurement criteria specific to informatics nurse specialists and their role and practice.

The standards of practice are organized using a general problem-solving framework that closely models the language provided in *Nursing: Scope and Standards of Practice* (ANA, 2004) that describes the familiar nursing process of assessment, diagnosis, identification of outcomes, planning, implementation, and evaluation. The problem-solving framework supports all facets of informatics practice, helps to identify and clarify issues, and aids in the selection, development, implementation, and evaluation of informatics solutions. These steps are not mutually exclusive and may often overlap.

Informatics solution is a generic term used in this document to describe an application, product, method, tool, workflow change, or other recommendation an informatics nurse makes after identifying and analyzing an issue. An informatics solution may encompass technology and non-technology elements such as developing a database, purchasing a new computer application, creating a standardized nursing vocabulary, designing informatics curricula, creating a spreadsheet, tailoring an application to a particular environment, designing a research study to describe required informatics competencies, describing information flow in a process redesign, creating newly re-engineered processes, or creating a structure for information presentation.

The standards of professional performance also reflect the model language provided in *Nursing: Scope and Standards of Practice* (ANA, 2004). They have been re-ordered, and include one additional standard that addresses advocacy.

These standards of nursing informatics practice and their measurement criteria apply to *all* informatics nurses and their practices. The measurement criteria for the informatics nurse specialist reflect the higher expectations from this role and advanced level of practice.

Principles of Nursing Informatics Practice

Three overarching principles are inherent in every aspect of nursing informatics practice and should be considered by informatics nurses and informatics nurse specialists when reviewing the standards of practice.

The informatics nurse:

1. Incorporates theories, principles, and concepts from appropriate sciences into informatics practice. Examples of theories could include information, systems, and change theories. Principles and concepts could include project management, implementation methods, workflow analysis, process redesign, organizational culture, or database structures.

2. Integrates ergonomics and human–computer interaction (HCI) principles into informatics solution design, development, selection, implementation, and evaluation.

3. Systematically determines the social, legal, regulatory, and ethical impact of an informatics solution on nursing and health care.

STANDARDS OF NURSING INFORMATICS
STANDARDS OF PRACTICE

STANDARD 1. ASSESSMENT
The informatics nurse collects comprehensive data, information, and knowledge pertinent to the situation.

Measurement Criteria:

The informatics nurse:

- Collects data, information, and knowledge in a systematic and on-going process, such as with a needs assessment to refine the issue or problem, or with workflow analyses to examine current practice, workflow, and the potential impact of an informatics solution on that workflow.

- Involves the patient, family, nurse, other healthcare providers, and key stakeholders, as appropriate, in holistic data collection.

- Prioritizes data collection activities based on the immediate or anticipated needs of the situation.

- Uses appropriate evidence-based assessment techniques and instruments in collecting pertinent data to define the issue or problem.

- Uses analytical models and assessment tools that facilitate problem solving.

- Synthesizes available data, information, and knowledge relevant to the situation to identify patterns and variances.

- Documents relevant data in a retrievable format.

STANDARD 2. PROBLEM AND ISSUES IDENTIFICATION
The informatics nurse analyzes the assessment data to determine the problems or issues.

Measurement Criteria:

The informatics nurse:

- Derives the problems, needs, or issues based on assessment data.

- Validates the problems, needs, or issues with the patient, family, nurse, other healthcare providers, and key stakeholders when possible and appropriate.

- Documents problems, needs, or issues in a manner that facilitates the determination of the expected outcomes and plan.

The content in this appendix is not current and is of historical significance only.

STANDARD 3. OUTCOMES IDENTIFICATION
The informatics nurse identifies expected outcomes for a plan individualized to the situation.

Measurement Criteria:

The informatics nurse:

- Involves the patient, family, nurses, other healthcare providers, and key stakeholders in formulating expected outcomes when possible and appropriate.

- Considers associated risks, benefits, costs, current scientific evidence, environmental factors, and expertise when formulating expected outcomes.

- Defines expected outcomes in terms of the patient, patient values, ethical considerations, environment, organization, or situation with such consideration as associated risks, benefits, and costs, and current evidence-based knowledge.

- Includes a time estimate for attainment of expected outcomes.

- Develops expected outcomes that provide direction for all key stakeholders.

- Modifies expected outcomes based on changes in the status or evaluation of the situation.

- Documents expected outcomes as measurable goals.

Additional Measurement Criteria for the Informatics Nurse Specialist:

The informatics nurse specialist:

- Identifies expected outcomes that incorporate scientific evidence and are achievable through implementation of evidence-based practices.

- Identifies expected outcomes that maximize quality, efficiency, and effectiveness balanced with economy.

- Supports the use of clinical guidelines, such as but not limited to the integration of clinical guidelines into practice, information system and informatics solutions, and knowledge bases.

The content in this appendix is not current and is of historical significance only.

STANDARD 4. PLANNING

The informatics nurse develops a plan that prescribes strategies, alternatives, and recommendations to attain expected outcomes.

Measurement Criteria:

The informatics nurse:

- Develops a customized plan considering clinical and business characteristics and the environmental situation.

- Develops the plan in conjunction with the patient, family, nurse, other healthcare providers, key stakeholders, and others, as appropriate.

- Includes strategies in the plan that address each of the identified problems and issues, which may include strategies for the synthesis of data, information, and knowledge to enhance healthcare delivery.

- Provides for continuity within the plan.

- Incorporates an implementation pathway or timeline within the plan.

- Establishes the plan priorities with the key stakeholders and others as appropriate.

- Utilizes the plan to provide direction to healthcare team members and other stakeholders.

- Defines the plan to reflect current statutes, rules and regulations, and quality standards.

- Integrates current research and trends in the planning process.

- Considers the clinical, financial, and social impact of the plan.

- Uses standardized language, tools, and methodologies to document the plan.

- Participates in the design and development of interdisciplinary processes and informatics principles to address the situation or issue.

- Contributes to the development and continuous improvement of organizational systems that support the planning process.

- Supports the integration of clinical, human, financial, and technical resources to enhance and complete the decision-making processes.

The content in this appendix is not current and is of historical significance only.

STANDARD 5. IMPLEMENTATION
The informatics nurse implements the identified plan.

Measurement Criteria:

The informatics nurse:

- Implements the plan in a safe and timely manner.

- Documents implementation and any modifications, including changes or omissions, of the identified plan.

- Utilizes specific evidence-based actions and steps specific to the problem or issues to achieve the defined outcomes.

- Utilizes clinical, financial, technical, and community resources and systems to implement the plan.

- Collaborates with colleagues and other stakeholders to implement the plan.

- Implements the plan using principles and concepts of quality, project, or systems management.

- Fosters organizational systems that support implementation of the plan.

- Incorporates new knowledge and strategies to initiate change in informatics and nursing practices if desired outcomes are not achieved.

STANDARD 5A: COORDINATION OF ACTIVITIES
The informatics nurse coordinates activities.

Measurement Criteria:

The informatics nurse:

- Coordinates implementation of the plan, including activities and resources necessary to achieve desired outcomes.

- Synthesizes data and information to prescribe necessary system and environmental support measures.

- Documents coordination of the activities.

Measurement Criteria for the Informatics Nurse Specialist:

The informatics nurse specialist:

- Provides leadership in the coordination of interdisciplinary informatics activities.

- Coordinates system and community resources that enhance delivery of care across continuums.

STANDARD 5B: HEALTH TEACHING AND HEALTH PROMOTION AND EDUCATION

The informatics nurse employs strategies to promote health teaching, health promotion, and education for informatics solutions.

Measurement Criteria:

The informatics nurse:

- Identifies the need to integrate health content and learning resources into healthcare systems that address such topics as healthy lifestyles, risk-reducing behaviors, developmental needs, activities of daily living, and preventive self-care.

- Participates in the design, development, implementation, and evaluation of health promotion materials and health teaching methods appropriate to the situation and the patient's developmental level, learning needs, readiness, ability to learn, language preference, and culture. The informatics nurse focuses on the integration of these into informatics solutions.

- Contributes to the design, development, implementation, and evaluation of the educational content, materials, and teaching strategies in a holistic manner (psychosocial, cognitive, affective) needed for the continuing education and professional development programs necessary to implement the plan.

Additional Measurement Criteria for the Informatics Nurses Specialist:

The informatics nurse specialist:

- Synthesizes empirical evidence on risk behaviors, learning theories, behavioral change theories, motivational theories, epidemiology, and other related theories and frameworks when designing health information and patient education materials and programs.

- Designs health information and patient education appropriate to the patient's developmental level, learning needs, readiness to learn, and cultural values and beliefs.

Continued ▶

The content in this appendix is not current and is of historical significance only.

- Evaluates health information resources, such as the Internet, within the area of practice for accuracy, readability, and comprehensibility to help patients, family, healthcare providers, and others access quality health information.

- Creates opportunities for feedback and evaluation of the effectiveness of the educational content and teaching strategies used for continuing education and professional development programs.

STANDARD 5C: CONSULTATION
The informatics nurse provides consultation to influence the identified plan, enhance the abilities of others, and effect change.

Measurement Criteria:

The informatics nurse:

- Synthesizes data, information, theoretical frameworks, and evidence when providing consultation.

- Facilitates the effectiveness of a consultation by involving the stakeholders in the decision-making process.

- Communicates consultation recommendations that influence the identified plan, facilitate understanding by involved stakeholders, enhance the work of others, and effect change.

Additional Measurement Criteria for the Informatics Nurses Specialist:

The informatics nurse specialist:

- Develops recommendations and strategies to address and resolve complex issues and problems.

- Establishes formal and informal consultative relationships that can also provide professional development and mentorship opportunities.

The content in this appendix is not current and is of historical significance only.

STANDARD 6. EVALUATION
The informatics nurse evaluates progress towards attainment of outcomes.

Measurement Criteria:

The informatics nurse:

- Conducts a systematic, ongoing, and criterion-based evaluation of the outcomes in relation to the structures and processes prescribed by the plan and the indicated timeline.

- Includes key stakeholders and others involved in the plan or situation in the evaluative process.

- Supports the integration and use of evidence-based methods, tools, and guidelines linked to effective outcomes.

- Evaluates the effectiveness of the planned strategies in relation to the attainment of the expected outcomes.

- Uses ongoing assessment data to revise the problems and issues, the outcomes, the plan, and the implementation and evaluative processes as needed.

- Disseminates the results to key stakeholders and others involved in the plan or situation as appropriate.

- Documents the results of the evaluation.

Additional Measurement Criteria for the Informatics Nurse Specialist:

The Informatics nurse specialist:

- Uses the results of the evaluation analyses to make or recommend process or structural changes including policy, procedure, or protocol documentation, as appropriate.

- Synthesizes the results of the evaluation analyses to determine the impact of the plan on the affected patients, families, groups, communities, and institutions, networks, and organizations.

STANDARDS OF PROFESSIONAL PERFORMANCE

STANDARD 7. EDUCATION
The informatics nurse attains knowledge and competency that reflect current nursing and informatics practice.

Measurement Criteria:

The informatics nurse:

- Participates in ongoing educational activities related to appropriate knowledge bases and professional issues.

- Demonstrates a commitment to lifelong learning through self-reflection and inquiry to identify learning needs.

- Seeks experiences that reflect current practice in order to maintain skills and competence in informatics practice and role performance.

- Acquires knowledge and skills appropriate to the specialty area, practice setting, role, or situation.

- Maintains professional records that provide evidence of competency and lifelong learning.

- Seeks experiences and formal and independent learning activities to maintain and develop clinical and professional skills and knowledge.

Additional Measurement Criteria for the Informatics Nurse Specialist:

The informatics nurse specialist:

- Uses current research findings and other evidence to expand knowledge, enhance role performance, and increase knowledge of professional issues.

The content in this appendix is not current and is of historical significance only.

STANDARD 8. PROFESSIONAL PRACTICE EVALUATION

The informatics nurse evaluates one's own nursing and informatics practice in relation to professional practice standards and guidelines, relevant statutes, rules, and regulations.

Measurement Criteria:

The informatics nurse's practice reflects the application of knowledge of current practice standards, guidelines, statutes, rules, and regulations.

The informatics nurse:

- Engages in self-evaluation of practice on a regular basis, identifying areas of strength as well as areas in which professional development would be beneficial.

- Obtains informal feedback regarding one's own practice from peers, professional colleagues, key stakeholders, and others.

- Participates in systematic peer review as appropriate.

- Takes action to achieve goals identified during the evaluation process.

- Provides rationales for practice beliefs, decisions, and actions as part of the informal and formal evaluation processes.

STANDARD 9. QUALITY OF PRACTICE
The informatics nurse systematically enhances the quality and effectiveness of nursing and informatics practice.

Measurement Criteria:

The informatics nurse:

- Demonstrates quality by documenting the application of the nursing process in a responsible, accountable, and ethical manner.

- Uses the results of quality improvement activities to initiate changes in nursing and informatics practice and in the healthcare delivery system.

- Uses creativity and innovation in nursing and informatics practice to improve care delivery.

- Incorporates new knowledge to initiate changes in nursing and informatics practice if desired outcomes are not achieved.

- Participates in quality improvement activities. Such activities may include:

  - Identifying aspects of practice important for quality monitoring.

  - Using indicators developed to monitor quality and effectiveness of nursing and informatics practice.

  - Collecting data to monitor quality and effectiveness of nursing and informatics practice.

  - Analyzing quality data to identify opportunities for improving nursing and informatics practice.

  - Formulating recommendations to improve nursing and informatics practice or outcomes.

  - Implementing activities to enhance the quality of nursing and informatics practice.

  - Engaging in the development, implementation, and evaluation of policies, procedures, and guidelines to improve the quality of practice.

Continued ▶

The content in this appendix is not current and is of historical significance only.

- - Participating on interdisciplinary teams to evaluate clinical care or delivery of health services.

  - Participating in efforts to minimize costs and unnecessary duplication.

  - Analyzing factors related to safety, satisfaction, effectiveness, and cost–benefit options.

  - Analyzing organizational systems for barriers.

  - Implementing processes to remove or decrease barriers within organizational systems.

- Obtains and maintains professional certification if available in the area of expertise.

- Designs quality improvement initiatives.

- Implements initiatives to evaluate the need for change.

- Evaluates the practice environment in relation to existing evidence, identifying opportunities for the generation and use of research.

STANDARD 10. COLLEGIALITY

The informatics nurse interacts with and contributes to the professional development of peers and colleagues.

Measurement Criteria:

The informatics nurse:

- Shares knowledge and skills with peers and colleagues as evidenced by such activities as presentations at formal or informal meetings and professional conferences.

- Provides peers with feedback regarding their practice and role performance.

- Interacts with peers and colleagues to enhance one's own professional nursing practice and role performance.

- Maintains compassionate and caring relationships with peers and colleagues.

- Contributes to an environment that is conducive to the education of healthcare professionals.

- Contributes to a supportive and healthy work environment.

Additional Measurement Criteria for the Informatics Nurse Specialist:

The informatics nurse specialist:

- Participates on interdisciplinary professional teams that contribute to role development and, directly or indirectly, advance nursing, informatics practice, and health services.

- Mentors other registered nurses and colleagues as appropriate.

The content in this appendix is not current and is of historical significance only.

STANDARD 11. COLLABORATION

The informatics nurse collaborates with key stakeholders and others in the conduct of nursing and informatics practice.

Measurement Criteria:

The informatics nurse:

- Communicates with key stakeholders regarding the practice of nursing and informatics.

- Communicates with key stakeholders regarding the role of nurses and nursing within the domain of healthcare informatics and patient care delivery.

- Collaborates in creating a documented plan focused on outcomes and decisions related to the management of data, information, and knowledge for the delivery of healthcare services.

- Partners with others to effect change and generate positive outcomes through knowledge of the plan and situation.

- Documents plans, communications, rationales for plan changes, and collaborative discussions.

Additional Measurement Criteria for Informatics Nurse Specialist:

The informatics nurse specialist:

- Partners with others to enhance health care, and ultimately patient care, through interdisciplinary activities such as education, consultation, management, technological development, or research opportunities.

The content in this appendix is not current and is of historical significance only.

STANDARD 12. ETHICS
The informatics nurse integrates ethical provisions in all areas of practice.

Measurement Criteria:

The informatics nurse:

- Uses *Code of Ethics for Nurses with Interpretive Statements* (ANA, 2001) to guide practice.

- Uses nursing and informatics principles and methodologies in a manner that preserves and protects patient autonomy, dignity, and rights.

- Employs informatics principles, standards, and methodologies to establish and maintain patient confidentiality within legal and regulatory parameters.

- Evaluates factors related to privacy, security, and confidentiality in the use and handling of data, information, and knowledge.

- Promotes active engagement of community members in the oversight and management of the exchange of health information.

- Serves as a patient advocate assisting patients in developing skills for self advocacy.

- Contributes to resolving ethical issues of patients, colleagues, or systems as evidenced in such activities as participating on ethics committees.

- Reports illegal, incompetent, or impaired practices.

- Seeks available resources as needed when formulating ethical decisions.

- Demonstrates a commitment to practicing self-care, managing stress, and connecting with self and others.

Continued ▶

The content in this appendix is not current and is of historical significance only.

Additional Measurement Criteria for the Informatics Nurse Specialist:

The informatics nurse specialist

- Participates on multidisciplinary and interdisciplinary teams that address ethical risks, benefits, and outcomes.

- Informs administrators or others of the risks, benefits, and outcomes of programs and decisions that affect healthcare delivery.

The content in this appendix is not current and is of historical significance only.

STANDARD 13. RESEARCH
The informatics nurse integrates research findings into practice.

Measurement Criteria:

The informatics nurse:

- Utilizes the best available evidence, including research findings, to guide practice decisions.

- Actively participates in research activities at various levels appropriate to the nurse's level of education and position. Such activities may include:

  - Identifying clinical, nursing, and informatics problems or issues specific to nursing research.

  - Participating in data collection such as surveys, pilot projects, and formal studies.

  - Participating in a formal committee or program.

  - Sharing research activities and findings with peers and others.

  - Conducting research.

  - Critically analyzing and interpreting research for application to practice.

  - Using research findings in the development of policies, procedures, and standards of practice in patient care.

  - Incorporating research as a basis for learning.

Additional Measurement Criteria for the Informatics Nurse Specialist:

The informatics nurse specialist:

- Contributes to nursing knowledge by conducting or synthesizing research that discovers, examines, and evaluates knowledge, theories, criteria, and creative approaches to improve health care.

- Formally disseminates research findings through activities such as presentations, publications, consultation, and journal clubs.

STANDARD 14. RESOURCE UTILIZATION

The informatics nurse considers factors related to safety, effectiveness, cost, and impact on practice in the planning and delivery of services to achieve expected outcomes.

Measurement Criteria:

The informatics nurse:

- Evaluates factors such as safety, effectiveness, availability, cost and benefits, efficiencies, and impact on practice, when choosing practice options that would result in the same expected outcome.

- Assists stakeholders in identifying and securing appropriate and available services to address identified needs and implement and complete the plan or other activity.

- Assigns or delegates tasks based on the knowledge, skills, and abilities of the individual, complexity of the task, and predictability of the outcome.

- Assists stakeholders in becoming informed consumers about the options, costs, risks, and benefits of the plan and its associated activities.

Additional Measurement Criteria for the Informatics Nurse Specialist:

The informatics nurse specialist:

- Develops innovative solutions and applies strategies to obtain appropriate resources for nursing initiatives.

- Secures organizational resources to ensure a work environment conducive to completing the identified plan and outcomes.

- Develops evaluation methods to measure the safety and effectiveness of interventions and outcomes.

- Promotes activities that assist stakeholders, as appropriate, in becoming informed about costs, risks, and benefits of care or of the plan and solution.

STANDARD 15. ADVOCACY

The informatics nurse advocates for the protections and rights of patients, healthcare providers, institutions and organizations, and for issues related to data, information, knowledge, and health care.

Measurement Criteria:

The informatics nurse:

- Supports patients' access to their own personal health information within a reasonable time.

- Promotes patients' awareness of how their personal health data and information may be used and who has access to it.

- Supports the individual's right and ability to supplement, request correction of, and share their personal health data and information.

- Evaluates factors related to privacy, security, and confidentiality in the use and handling of health information.

- Promotes awareness and education of the healthcare consumer with regard to appropriate data collection, information sharing, information access, and associated issues.

- Supports patient involvement in their own care, facilitated by access to personal healthcare data.

- Promotes active engagement of community members in the development, oversight, and management of health information exchange.

- Educates clinicians, patients, and communities about the rights, responsibilities, and accountability entailed in the collection, use, and exchange of healthcare data and information.

- Incorporates the identified needs of the patient, family, healthcare provider, organization, and key stakeholders in policy development, program and services planning, and systems design.

- Integrates advocacy into the implementation of policies, programs and services, and systems for the patient.

Continued ▶

The content in this appendix is not current and is of historical significance only.

- Evaluates the effectiveness of advocating for the patient, family, healthcare provider, organization, and key stakeholders when assessing the actual outcomes.

- Demonstrates skill in advocating before providers and stakeholders on behalf of the patient, community, or population.

- Strives to resolve conflicting expectations from patients, families, communities, populations, healthcare providers, and other stakeholders.

Additional Measurement Criteria for the Informatics Nurse Specialist:

The informatics nurse specialist:

- Demonstrates skill in advocating on behalf of the patient, key stakeholders, programs, and services before public representatives and decision-makers.

- Exhibits fiscal responsibility and integrity in advocacy and formulating policy.

- Serves as an expert for patients, peers, other healthcare providers, and other stakeholders in promoting and implementing policies related to the management of data, information, and knowledge.

Standard 16. Leadership
The informatics nurse provides leadership in the professional practice setting and the profession.

Measurement Criteria:

The informatics nurse:

- Engages in teamwork as a team player and a team builder.

- Works to create and maintain healthy work environments in local, regional, national, or international communities.

- Displays the ability to define a clear vision, the associated goals, and a plan to implement and measure progress.

- Demonstrates a commitment to continuous, lifelong learning for self and others.

- Teaches others to succeed by mentoring and other strategies.

- Exhibits creativity and flexibility through times of change.

- Demonstrates energy, excitement, and a passion for quality work.

- Willingly accepts mistakes by self and others, thereby creating a culture in which risk-taking is not only safe, but expected.

- Inspires loyalty through valuing of people as the most precious asset in an organization.

- Directs the coordination of the plan across settings and among caregivers and other stakeholders.

- Serves in key roles in the work setting by participating on committees, councils, and administrative teams.

- Promotes advancement of the profession through participation in professional organizations.

- Assumes leadership roles within organizations representing nursing informatics professional practice in the healthcare domain.

Continued ▶

The content in this appendix is not current and is of historical significance only.

Additional Measurement Criteria for the Informatics Nurse Specialist:

The informatics nurse specialist:

- Serves in key leadership roles defining the vision, strategy, and tactical plans related to the management of data, information, and knowledge.

- Works to influence decision-making bodies to improve patient care, health services, and policies through such things as the adoption of data standards.

- Promotes communication of information and advancement of the profession through writing, publishing, and presentations for professional or lay audiences.

- Designs innovations to effect change in practice and outcomes.

- Provides direction to enhance the effectiveness of the interdisciplinary team and key stakeholders.

Index

An index entry preceded by a bracketed calendar year indicates an entry from a previous edition or predecessor publication that is included in this edition as an appendix.

F

K

KDD (knowledge discovery in databases), 21

Knowledge and NI practice
defined, 3
evidence-based practice and, 83
NI competencies and, 47
as NI metastructure, 2–6
[2008], 116–118, 126
representation trends, 59
[2008], 167
as synthesis of data and information,
3, 4, 7, 21
Wisdom-in-Action for Clinical
Nursing© model, 107
See also Metastructures, concepts,
and tools of NI; Wisdom and NI
practice

Knowledge base. *See* Body of knowledge

Knowledge discovery in databases
(KDD), 21, 59
[2008], 132–133

L

Laws, statutes, and regulations
assessment and, 69
changes, trends in, 62–63
ethics and, 79
[2008], 196
information systems life cycle, 18–19
[2008], 131
planning and, 72
[2008], 183
problems and issues identification
[2008], 181
professional practice evaluation
and, 91
[2008], 191
See also Ethics

Leadership
coordination of activities and, 75
[2008], 185
as functional area in NI, 18–21
[2008], 131–132

standard of professional performance,
87–88
[2008], 202–203
See also Mentoring

Leapfrog, 62

Learning management system (LMS), 25

Licensed practical nurse (LPN), 42

Licensing. *See* Certification and
credentialing

LMS (learning management system), 25

Logical Observation Identifiers, Names,
and Codes (LOINC®), 10, 13

LOINC® (Logical Observation
Identifiers, Names, and Codes), 10, 13

M

Machine learning methods, 21

Management as functional area in NI,
18–21
[2008], 131–132

Matney, Susan, 107

Measurement criteria for NI practice
[2008], 180–203
advocacy [2008], 200–201
assessment [2008], 180
collaboration [2008], 195
collegiality [2008], 194
consultation [2008], 188
coordination of activities [2008],
185
education [2008], 190
ethics [2008], 196–197
evaluation [2008], 189
health teaching and health promotion
and education [2008], 186–187
implementation [2008], 184
leadership [2008], 202–203
outcomes identification [2008], 182
planning [2008], 183
problem and issues identification
[2008], 181
professional practice evaluation
[2008], 191